Stir

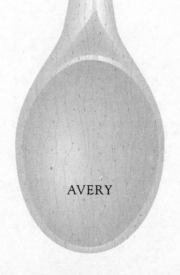

stir

MY BROKEN BRAIN
AND THE MEALS
THAT BROUGHT
ME HOME

Jessica Fechtor

AVERY

An imprint of Penguin Random House
375 Hudson Street
New York, New York 10014

Some of the recipes and brief portions of this book appeared in different form on the author's blog, Sweet Amandine.

Portions of chapter 30 were originally published in slightly different form in *Tablet Magazine* (www.tabletmag.com).

Excerpt from *Omeros* by Derek Walcott. Copyright © 1990 by Derek Walcott. Reprinted by permission of Farrar, Straus and Giroux, LLC.

Most Avery books are available at special quantity discounts for bulk purchase for sales promotions, premiums, fund-raising, and educational needs. Special books or book excerpts also can be created to fit specific needs. For details, write Special.Markets@penguinrandomhouse.com

LIBRARY OF CONGRESS CATALOGING-IN-PUBLICATION DATA
Fechtor, Jessica.
Stir : my broken brain and the meals that brought me home / Jessica Fechtor.
pages cm
ISBN 978-1-59463-132-0
1. Fechtor, Jessica—Health.   2. Intracranial aneurysms—Patients—United States—Biography.   3. Intracranial aneurysms—Patients—Rehabilitation—United States.   4. Cooking—Therapeutic use.   I. Title.
RC693.F43 2015
616.1'330092—dc23
[B]
                                                                    2014048572

Printed in the United States of America

10   9   8   7   6   5   4   3   2   1

Set in Goudy Oldstyle Std   ·   Designed by Eve Kirch

For Mom, Dad, and Amy

And for Eli, of course

Measure the days you have left. Do just that labour
which marries your heart to your right hand: simplify
your life to one emblem, a sail leaving harbour
and a sail coming in. . . .

—DEREK WALCOTT, *Omeros*

Contents

Stir

Prologue

I am on the floor.

My back is flat against the ground, and so are the soles of my feet, and my knees are up and swaying. Someone is holding my head at the temples. "Jessica, it's Ilana." She says it the Canadian way, with a flat first *a. Lavish, lamb, Atlantic.*

My knees are swaying.

I turn my head and vomit into her lap. The hotel gym guy comes with orange Gatorade. He is tall and waxy with a bird face and dark hair that's more thin than thinning. He wants to know if I've had any breakfast. "A banana," I tell him, and he nods as though he suspected as much. He bends at the waist and wags the bottle over my face for me to take it. I vomit again. Ilana doesn't flinch.

I'm at a graduate student conference in Stowe, Vermont, a town wedged deep in the valley between the Green Mountains and the Worcester Range. I am twenty-eight years old. Ilana is a colleague. I've seen her at these conferences over the last couple of years, and we've shared meals, but that's all. I'm grateful for the pad of her thigh.

I see my friend Or. We'd planned to run together along the country roads that morning, but a crack of thunder had sent us to the gym instead. He stands over me now in a tank top with a bandana tied low across his forehead. He looks like a pirate and says he's going to call. The gym guy insists it's not necessary, but Or calls.

An ambulance is coming.

It's August and the sky is dark from the storm. I don't try to get up. I don't even think to try—it will be years before I realize the oddness of that—and no one offers to help me. Ilana is talking to me, and Or is talking to me, and Or and Ilana are talking to each other about me, and the girl who was on the treadmill next to mine is talking to someone, the gym guy maybe, about "what happened." I can hear the spit moving around in her mouth as she speaks. She sounds breathless and scared and I want her to be quiet. Someone at the opening session the night before had mentioned that he was training as an EMT and they bring him in. He looks me in the eye, expressionless, then steps away.

My knees are swaying.

I've had migraines before. The pain feels similar, so I assume that's what this is. I've never fainted, though, and it has never come on so fast. A flash migraine, then. *Is that a thing?* I can't decide if I'm supposed to be scared.

Or is asking me whom he should call and I tell him my dad, no, Eli. I give him my husband's number and watch him dial. My head hurts so badly, and I think that if I can relax my body, get really quiet, I can make it better. Ilana says, "She's not talking anymore."

The paramedic arrives. He shines lights and asks if I remember the fall, and I do.

I was running on the treadmill, when I felt a painless click in my head. There was an odd trickling sensation along my skull like a rolling bead of sweat, but on the inside. Then the room went gray and the earth sucked me down. I knew I was about to faint. The red stop button seemed suddenly far away. I swiped at it, but there was no time to step off the machine. Someone says I hit my head on the way down, and I wonder if the belt was still moving when I fell. I can no longer sway my knees; the paramedic's in the way, so I start rubbing his leg instead.

"I'm sorry," I say, "I'm rubbing your leg."

"That's all right. You keep rubbing."

He tells me to fold my arms across my chest, that they are going to strap me to a board and carry me to the ambulance. It's very important, he says, to call out if I need to vomit so that they can flip me over in time. The thought of that, of hanging facedown in the air and vomiting, the thought of being dropped, is at this moment the most terrifying thing in the world.

I start this story here, on the floor of a conference center gym, because it now seems the most obvious place. But it wasn't obvious to me then that a start had occurred at all. I thought my fall from the treadmill was a dot on a plotline already under way, the one about the literature student at a conference who fainted, missed the morning's events, got checked out, and returned, red faced and sheepish, in time for lunch. I didn't know then that when I slipped from that moving belt, that dot had also slipped and become its own point A.

What a click in my head, and a moving belt, and a headache that knocked me down might have to do with butter, and flour, and eggs at room temp, and hunger, and love, and a kitchen with something to say, I couldn't have known that day. How a detour could become its own path, I would never have believed.

Please Buy an Oven Thermometer

(Some Thoughts on Cooking from This Book)

So, yes, this is a book about food. It isn't a cookbook, though there are recipes here. Because to follow the story where it went I had to follow it into my kitchen. The recipes in this book are for foods that connect me to myself and to my people. Foods that reminded me who I was when I felt least like myself. My recipes are, for the most part, simple and straightforward, because that's the way I like to cook and eat. They're recipes that show you how to make food that feels special not because it's fancy, but because it tastes so good. I'm excited to share them with you.

We all have our ways in the kitchen. Before we get started, I want to tell you about some of mine. Think of it as preemptive troubleshooting, reducing the variables so that at your house, things just work. Of course, over time, I hope you'll make these recipes your own, with whatever tweaks and changes you see fit.

First, let's talk about measurements. I like to cook and, especially, bake by weight because I find it easier and faster, with more consistent results. A basic digital scale will do the trick; you don't need any bells or whistles. You can pick one up for around twenty dollars. Most household kitchen scales are not sensitive enough to reliably measure weights under ten grams. Any ingredient that measures under ¼ cup, I've listed by volume alone, in teaspoons and tablespoons.

Flour is especially tricky to measure by volume, since even the same cook measuring the same flour with the same cup can get considerable variation from scoop to scoop. It all depends on how tightly you pack your cup. If you don't have a scale or prefer to measure by volume, here's how to do it so that your amounts are closest to mine: Stir your jar or sack of flour with a fork to aerate it, spoon the flour into your measuring cup, and, without tapping the measuring cup to settle its contents, sweep the excess flour from the top with the straight back of a knife. The recipes in this book were tested with both weight and volume measurements by a small army of home cooks, cookbook authors, professional bakers, food bloggers, and food magazine editors, so either way, you should be set.

While we're on the subject of flour: For all-purpose unbleached white flour, I use the King Arthur brand. It has a higher protein content than other national brands (and a consistent protein content, bag to bag, which I appreciate). Protein content is relevant because more protein means more gluten development, and more water absorption when you combine it with your wet ingredients. That affects texture. King Arthur all-purpose flour contains about 12 percent protein. If you bake the cookies in this book using a brand that contains only, say, 9 percent protein, you can expect a wetter dough that will result in flatter, paler cookies with less chew. A higher-protein all-purpose flour like King Arthur is nice to have around because it also works well in breads. Convenient if you'd rather not purchase an additional sack of bread flour or don't have any on hand.

I use large eggs and unsalted butter when making the recipes in this book. I bake with fine-grain sea salt. You can use table salt instead, if that's what you've got. A few of the recipes in this book call for Diamond Crystal brand kosher salt. The brand is important because the size of the crystals varies among kosher salt brands. Morton's, for example, has a finer grain, so a teaspoon will be considerably saltier than a teaspoon of Diamond Crystal. If you swap in fine-grain sea salt or another brand of kosher salt for the Diamond Crystal, you'll need to use less. Taste as you go and trust your preferences.

A few of the recipes call for canned tomatoes or sauce. My preferred brand is Muir Glen. I always have a can or two of their organic whole peeled tomatoes in the cupboard, the tomatoes that, incidentally, beat out even the celebrated San Marzano tomatoes in a *Cook's Illustrated* taste test.

Last but not least, please buy an oven thermometer. Ovens, even shiny new ones, run hot and cold all the time. Some, like mine, overshoot by fifty degrees before settling back down to the temperature on the dial. It's not only a matter of under- or overbaking. Cakes, cookies, and breads baked at the wrong temperature will have issues with texture, too. It's the simplest thing, but an oven thermometer can make all the difference in what comes out of your kitchen.

Onward.

CHAPTER 1

The Pit

They say that trauma functions like a merciful eraser, wiping away into dust what the body most needs to forget. That's not how it worked for me. I remember all of it: the shifting hum of the treadmill as I cranked up the speed; feeling strong and fast until, in an instant, I wasn't. It was as though someone had tossed a giant lead cape over my shoulders. My knees bent too deeply. My eyelids drooped. "No, no," I breathed as I went down, my voice a note too high.

I'd never played sports as a kid and only started running after college. I liked the phrase "recreational runner" and thought it might be nice to be one, to "squeeze in a run" during lunch or "take a loop around the park" after work, like the people I knew who said those things. Turned out running was the perfect sport for my bookish, unathletic self. I loved the little goals, the on-your-own-ness of it. There was stuff to keep track of: miles, pace, nutrition. I got to have a notebook. For data!

Running is about putting one foot in front of the other to get where you want to be. It felt similar to my academic work in that way, the incremental progress, the stamina involved, but instead of a brain swollen with languages and texts, I got fitness. It was simple: By running, I was choosing health. I was certain I had a say.

The hotel room was dark when I woke up that morning. My roommate, Adena, was still sleeping, so I slipped on my running shorts and T-shirt as silently as I could. Or and I had planned to meet in the lobby and knock out six miles before breakfast. At the conference the year before, Or had invited me to join him on a run, but I had said no. He was a "real" runner, a marathoner, over six feet tall and strong. Running with him was way out of my league. But I'd been training all year, adding distance and speed. I'd just completed my first half marathon. With that under my belt, I felt brave enough to join him.

I don't like to think about what might have happened if there had been no storm that morning and we'd been out on the roads as planned, several miles from the conference center, without cell phones, in rural Vermont. But of course, I sometimes do think about it, and while I don't believe in fate, I do believe in very good luck and thank my stars for the rain that kept us back.

It had been a while since I'd traded a run outdoors for a treadmill. With the belt pulling itself out from under my feet with every stride, it felt easy. I like to let my thoughts take off on their own when I run, and meet them wherever they land: *Emancipation of serfs, 1861, under Alexander the Second. Assassinated, 1881.* It was three weeks before my first two doctoral exams, one on Russian history and one on Yiddish language. Twenty days, actually, so less. I'd have to renew that library book again. Or just buy it already.

All my exams would be done by Thanksgiving. I'd start my dissertation. Then, a baby, we hoped. *A baby.* I loved that Eli and I had come to it together, that wanting to be parents hadn't been a given for either of us when we married, at twenty-five, but that nearly three years later, we felt ready. I'd been off the pill for two weeks.

Eli and I had spent the summer in New York City. We'd swapped apartments with friends. Theirs was a two-room flat on East Third and Avenue A, two blocks from Katz's Deli in the heart of the Lower East Side. A few blocks in the other direction was St. Marks Place, home to an all-star plate of grilled haloumi and fried eggs. Due west was the Hudson River, and the path alongside it that goes all the way up the island. On Sunday mornings, I'd wake up early and run long, west to the highway, then north along the water eight, nine, ten miles, whatever my training plan prescribed. Then brunch at Café Mogador for those eggs.

Eli worked from our adopted home each day, designing software and finishing up a public art piece with a friend. I took Yiddish classes at NYU and prepared for my doctoral exams. Something was shifting for us that summer. We were on the cusp of something, and we felt it. We made a plan for our return to Cambridge: I'd knock out my exams. Eli would look for a tech job out west. We'd move in the spring. I would begin writing my dissertation on the fellowship I had already secured while, with any luck, a human started growing in my belly.

Our last night in New York we took ourselves out to an Italian wine bar on East Fourth. It was small and cavelike, with exposed brick walls and glowing naked bulbs hanging from the ceiling. The host led us to a corner table at the very front of the house and swung the giant casement windows open over the street. I sat with my back to them, propped my elbows on the sill, and leaned into the warm night air.

There was shaved fennel salad, fried artichokes, and porcini ravioli to share. We drank wine. Earlier that day, I told Eli, I'd mistakenly referred to him as "my boyfriend." It had just slipped out. But it still felt that way sometimes, didn't it? That he was my new boyfriend and I was his girl? We'd been together six years, married half as long, but it felt as though we'd just made that leap, half toppling, half sailing from the solid ground of our friendship into something new. He knew what I meant, he said. Nothing seemed to age us.

The next day we packed up our car, spent a long weekend with his family in New Jersey, and drove home to our one-bedroom in Cambridge, Massachusetts. It had felt good to be back in my kitchen again after a summer away, to stand at my counter squeezing tomato slabs and mayo between the familiar slices of a baguette from down the block. I set our table with the napkins we never bothered to iron and burned almonds in the oven I'd forgotten ran hot. I did some baking, too, just for fun, then parceled things out to our neighbors. Drop biscuits, a berry crisp, chocolate chip cookies. I was home.

They slid me from the ambulance at the small hospital in Stowe and hoisted me up on shoulders again. My face felt too close to the ceiling. I was embarrassed by the drama I'd kicked up around me. Surely, if I were sick, it was a wimpy little sick. Dehydration, maybe? Low blood sugar? And if this were something worse, we were on it. *We.* Ilana had kneeled at my head; Or had called 911; a paramedic had come. Cindy, on faculty at the conference, had ridden with me in the ambulance, up front. Adena, my friend and conference roommate, was on her way. These people would keep me safe. *I* would keep me safe, by the simple act of marching thoughts across my brain.

Up on the stretcher, I kept nodding off the way you do on an airplane or long road trip. The pain was excruciating, the drifting in and out of consciousness almost pleasant. I remember the room we entered, the doughnut-shaped machine, the technician, and how his gray curls and deep-set eyes made me feel he was up to the task. I don't remember the ride that followed to Fletcher Allen hospital in Burlington, a Level I trauma center equipped to handle what he saw: There was blood in my brain. And not neatly inside the vessels, where it's supposed to be. There had been a spill.

Cindy and Adena sat to the left of my stretcher in the Fletcher Allen ER. Machines beeped on my right. The beige curtain pulled closed around us parted and a grave-looking doctor stepped in, held out a clipboard, and asked me to sign. I was overcome with the desire to do a Very Good Job. The pen felt cool in my hand. I wrote my name slowly, as carefully as I could: *Jessica Kate Fechtor.* I was still wearing my workout clothes, the same Adidas shorts on the same legs that had carried me through the New York City half marathon a few weeks before. Cindy peeled the clothes from my clammy body and helped me into a gown.

"Hello, lady."

I looked up. Eli was there.

He was in his standard uniform, jeans and a black cotton tee, and was digging around near the machines looking for a place to plug in his phone. No luck, I guess, because he was back up now, darting around the foot of the bed, crouching on the other side.

His phone was dead. It had died at the start of his drive, just after he'd heard from Cindy, when no one knew anything at all. He'd spent the better part of four hours pushing a hundred miles per hour, distracting himself with the thought that it was kind of cool to have an excuse to drive that fast, rather than dwelling on what might be going on with me. When his mind did wander to what was waiting for him at the end of that trip, he imagined a supremely embarrassed Jess laughing with him at this big, noisy fuss over nothing.

He disappeared to the other side of the curtain and sneaked his phone charger into the USB port of a nurse's computer when no one was looking. I needed him to stop moving, sit down, give me his hand. But I also needed him not to, to keep being the speck of normal in a scene that made no sense.

A resident appeared. Young, serious, handsome. I trusted him right away. I assumed he was mine, *my doctor*, as though I'd have only one and he'd shepherd me through whatever happened. He confirmed that, yes, there was a hemorrhage. I had blood in my brain. They just weren't sure where it had come from. I asked him if I could die, and he looked me in the eye and said yes.

Well, as long as they know, I thought. As long as the worst possible thing was on their radar, they'd be able to ward it off. I assumed the doctor's "yes" had come with a silent clause: "Yes, if you weren't under our care." "Yes, you might have, but now you're here."

The ICU was ready for me. All the rooms were full, so they wheeled me into a large, brightly lit room with floors like the ones in my middle school cafeteria. Beds were perpendicular against the wall with curtains drawn around them, little islands of sick. I got a corner slot, all the way down on the left. Two nurses were there, smoothing the sheets, drawing back the curtain. They lit up when they saw me, as though they'd been expecting me, and maybe I'd been running late, and they were so happy I was finally there. They waved and smiled and said hello.

The nurse with the long red hair was Patty. She reached out both arms to me, and I felt suddenly quite happy to see them, too. It helped that their faces betrayed not a wink of pity or fear. They had the stance of people about to take very good care of me, but more in the way of hosts looking after their houseguests than nurses tending to the ill. Patty welcomed me to "the Pit" in a faux dramatic voice and smiled. That was what the nurses called this room where the overflow ICU patients stayed, she explained. I liked being in on the joke. I felt well enough to scoot from the stretcher to the bed myself, and I did. I threw up. Patty rubbed my back. I was sure it would all be okay.

CHAPTER 2

A Cake

When I tell people that I am writing the story of a bloodied and broken brain—and oh, by the way, there will be recipes, too—I get some strange looks. Food is not supposed to top the list of things you think about, apparently, when you're recovering from a near-fatal brain explosion. The thing is, I did think about food. A lot.

And it's not really all that strange. Thinking about food means thinking about everything that goes on around it. The dash from the breakfast table out the door, the conversations that shape us, the places and faces that make us who we are. What besides food could I think of that would encompass my life so roundly?

Illness takes away plenty of big things. You can't work; you can't play. Worst of all, though, is the way it robs you of your everyday. That's true whether you're sick for three months or three days. If you've ever had a shower after a fever breaks, a first bite of solid food, traded your bathrobe for your favorite sweater, then you've felt it, too. Getting well means finding your everyday. I found mine in the kitchen.

In the years before I got sick, I spent a lot of time in there. Kitchen business is physical. That was important to me during my first, healthy years of graduate school. After swimming around and around in my brain all day long, looping through the library after each paragraph written or chapter read so that I could remember what my legs were for, I wanted nothing more than to rub butter into flour, to feel the mild burn in my wrists and dough between my fingertips. I brought cakes to seminars, soups to neighbors, and mailed biscotti to faraway friends. I talked about food with anyone who would listen. I wrote about it, too: in the margins of my research notebooks, the pages of my journal, and summertime missives sent from study programs abroad.

Food has powers. It picks us up from our lonely corners and sits us back down, together. It pulls us out of ourselves, to the kitchen, to the table, to the diner down the block. At the same time, it draws us inward. Food is the keeper of our memories, connecting us with our pasts and with our people. A parsnip, for me, is Friday nights. It's a soup pot simmering with a chicken inside, silk curtains, and my grandmother smelling brothy, salted, and sweet.

But there's also something simpler going on, I think, namely that it feels so good to eat. Because we're hungry, yes, but also because food allows us, in some small way, to act out who we are. My aunt puts cream in her ginger ale. I put peanut butter on a spoon. And cottage cheese on baked potatoes, and milk in tea, and yogurt on top of granola, not the other way around. My brother has a recipe: "Mustard. Bread. Mustard sandwich." Eli comes from a family that puts ketchup on pasta and fries French toast in oil. He cuts off the crusts and saves them for last and eats them like bread sticks, with jam.

Food—like art, like music—brings people together, it's true. It begins, though, with a private experience, a single person stirred, moved, and wanting company in that altered state. So we say, "You have to taste this." We say, "Please, take a bite."

It is a pleasure not only to taste, but to have taste, to feel our preferences exert themselves. It feels good to know what we like, because that's how we know who we are.

I was born in New York City. My parents weren't "foodies" in the all-too-narrow sense we think of when we hear that word today, but lovers of food in the broadest, most democratic way. My mother gets excited over a glop of fruit-on-the-bottom yogurt and bran flakes. My father has been known to extol the virtues of a Nestlé Chunky bar. You see what I mean. They are, in the words of Calvin Trillin, "serious eaters," which, if you ask me, is a much more fitting way of describing people who have a thing for food. They don't eat terribly much or make any big deal about it. They just eat what they like and like what they eat. It's a matter of enthusiasm, really, a way of being that they took with them out into their city—to the hot dog stand, the ice cream counter, the kosher deli—and in so doing, taught me to do the same.

I baked with my mother when I was young. Butter cookies, brownies. "Don't forget to keep it in the bowl," she'd say as I stirred. But more important than anything I might have learned in the kitchen, what I inherited was a way of thinking about food, an openness to it, a hunger for it in all its forms.

We lived in a two-room apartment at Seventy-fifth and Third, my mother, my father, a cat named Spike, a shih tzu named Cheeseburger, and a baby me. It was a squeeze, so the functional took priority. The coffee table converted to dining height. The sofa pulled into a bed. That was where my parents slept, in the living-room-dining-room-turned-second-bedroom, when I was born and took over the only room with a door. "We were getting our money together," my mother once told me. They were getting their lives together.

My great-great-aunt Frances lived a few blocks away in an apartment three times the size. My memory of it begins in the living room, enormous and bright, with east-facing windows and bookcases that stretched floor to ceiling along the entire northern wall. In the dining room was a long table and, according to my mother, a buzzer on the floor that Aunt Fran would press with her foot to signal the housekeeper to bring the next course. If I'd eaten many meals in that room, I'd surely have remembered that, but I ate mostly in her kitchen, on a green vinyl stool with two steps up that folded out from beneath the seat cushion.

Rosemary, the housekeeper, slept in the adjoining room, and the kitchen was her domain. It took me years to understand that the cooking and cleaning Rosemary did was her job. As far as I could tell, she and Aunt Fran were roommates, Rosemary living there and helping as she did because Aunt Fran was old, not because she was paid to. It seemed a lovely thing to do.

Anyway, it was Rosemary who would seat me on that stool, tie a clean white dish towel around my neck, and hold out a bowl of bean-flecked vanilla ice cream with a grown-up-sized spoon. I can't quite picture Rosemary's face, but I remember a neat hairline and soft arms. I didn't yet know about the herb called rosemary, so her name made me think of roses instead.

Rosemary died when I was six, and when my parents told me, I cried. I wasn't sure if I had a right to, but I think now of something the British chef Nigel Slater once wrote, that it is "impossible not to love someone who makes toast for you." I think the same can be said of the person who scoops your ice cream into a dish and stands, smiling, as you eat.

We saw Aunt Fran all the time, but each visit felt like an occasion. She was my first old person, a pale woman with dark hair that hung to just below her ears. I can picture her charging down the sidewalk toward me, her trench coat billowing behind her like a cape, my mother doing her full-arm wave, as though trying to get the attention of someone not staring right at us.

Aunt Fran never had children, and by some standards you might say that she didn't know how to be with them. I thought she was great. Instead of talking to me in the labored way people sometimes do to bridge the adult-child divide, she operated as though there weren't one. Her voice was raspy and low, her eyes bright behind huge plastic frames. She would wait for me to speak, with a faint grin on her closed lips, then smile widely, with teeth, when I was through. She was observing me and, yes, judging, but only because she was listening for real.

I have a memory of sitting with Aunt Fran and my parents at a low table in a candlelit, wood-paneled restaurant. The white linens are crisp, and a waiter sails by with a plate of something delicate and dark. Aunt Fran points and tells me they're snails. She says it matter-of-factly; not how grown-ups sometimes say this kind of thing to children—*what do you make of that!*—but just to let me know. I am four years old and I do not flinch. She orders me escargots, and they arrive with a tiny fork, and no one makes a fuss, and I eat.

It's funny how the foods that inhabit our childhoods turn around to house our childhoods when we're grown. Snails, vanilla ice cream, minestrone from a can. I come from these things. From the croissants my mother would pull from white paper bags, tear in half, and stuff with Smucker's grape jelly, from her omelets, oozing with American cheese, from tiny amaretti that came in a red square tin. A babysitter first brought them over, and though there was nothing special that I can remember about that night, those amaretti made an impression. The tins, with their Italian lettering and fleurs-de-lis, made the cookies seem fancy, but really they weren't. They were just bite-sized buttons of egg whites and sugar, flavored with apricot kernels. I had a vague sense that being grown-up meant appreciating a thing like that, a thing so simple. And while being grown-up was not necessarily something to which I aspired, I enjoyed being a kid who appreciated grown-up things.

When I was five, my family moved from New York to Ohio, just east of Cleveland, and I brought the empty tin with me. The scent of the cookies clung to it for years. Sometimes I'd lie on my bed beneath the sloped ceiling of our farmhouse, pry open the lid, and inhale. It triggered not so much a memory as an awareness of something I'd forgotten. Eventually, I forgot the tin, too.

Fifteen years later, I was home from college on winter break. And by "home" I don't mean that farmhouse where my parents, baby sister, and I had lived; nor, God forbid, the apartment with green shag carpeting my father moved into two years later when my parents split; nor the contemporary suburban home where my mother, sister, and I moved a few years after that; nor any of the houses where my father lived with his new wife and, within a couple of years of their marriage, two new kids.

This home was in Bexley, a suburb of Columbus, Ohio. My father and his family had settled there before their kids were school age and stayed, and because most of my people lived there, it felt like my home, too. I entered the house through the side door that winter and dropped my bags. I smelled it before I saw it. The toasted nuts, the floral note of the almond extract, the butter. It sat in a fluted tart pan beneath a veil of sliced almonds and sugar.

A cake.

My stepmother, Amy, had baked it for later that night. There had been no occasion, just a recipe from the paper she'd wanted to try, which for her is occasion enough. The recipe is as simple as they come: just sugar, butter, eggs, flour, and salt, with a splash each of vanilla and almond extract. It's a rich cake with a tender crumb, dense and delicate at the same time, humble despite its fluting. From its aroma alone, I knew that it was somehow mine, and when I took a bite, I knew why: *Those cookies. Those amaretto cookies.*

It was a clown car of a cake. My aunt Fran was in there, her coat flapping in the wind, our city street, and a rush of warm air forced up through the subway grates. A block party in Brooklyn where the big kids drank soda, the backseat of a taxi, a playground tire swing, my parents, hand in hand. Amaretto is made from apricot kernels, not almonds, but something about the way that cake looked, how it smelled, how it tasted, how it felt, how *I* felt, home from college with it on my plate—that old sense of being small but grown-up, that new sense of being grown-up but still small—bridged the flavors in my mind.

That cake was, in many ways, where it all started for me, this awareness that food is more than food. It got me thinking about the kind of baker and cook I wanted to be, made me understand that food had something to tell me, and that it felt good to listen.

In the nine years between that cake and when I got sick, my food told me a lot. I learned that when you put freshly baked bread and a lump of softened butter on the table, you are taking good care of your people, no matter the rest of the meal. You can serve that still-warm bread with a day-old salad or a plate of apple wedges, a can of beans, or a simple cup of tea. Your people will feel fed. I learned that a bowl full of mango, fully skinned, pit removed, and sliced into slippery cubes, is pure love. Same goes for a bowl of supremed oranges, all the pith stripped away, vesicles exposed like jewels.

Best of all, I learned to pay attention. I learned to watch people, how they eat, what they do with their bodies, their faces, their voices and their words, when they sit down at my table. I know, for example, that my friend Eitan will always reach for the bread I've brushed with egg white and sprinkled with oats, while my sister Kasey prefers the one with the sunflower and pumpkin seeds. She'll press her finger onto her plate at the end of the meal to get the stray ones. I know that my mother gets a kick out of a fried egg on her salad, that my father slaps the table when he takes a bite of sautéed kale, that Eli likes his apple cake with more apples, and that I do, too. When I piece together a menu for a tableful of family and friends, I think about all these things. From my hospital bed, far from that table, I did, too.

Marcella's Butter Almond Cake

This is the almond cake that met me that night in Ohio. It's my secret weapon in the kitchen, one of those cakes that comes together in no time from practically nothing, but is so pretty and tastes so good that no one ever believes you. Amy got the recipe from her friend Patricia, who clipped it from *The Columbus Dispatch*, and I've adapted it here. For short, Amy and I call this cake "Marcella's" after its creator, Marcella Sarne, who entered it in a baking contest sponsored by C&H Sugar and won, to the tune of a grand-prize custom kitchen.

My friend Janet suggests sprinkling a pinch of salt over the batter together with the toasted almonds and sugar. My friend Janet, by the way, is a genius. Covered and stored at room temperature, this cake keeps well for several days.

Butter and flour for the pan
3 heaped tablespoons sliced almonds
¾ cup (1½ sticks; 170 grams) unsalted butter, melted and slightly cooled
1½ cups (300 grams) granulated sugar, plus 1 tablespoon for finishing
2 large eggs
1½ teaspoons pure almond extract
1½ teaspoons pure vanilla extract
¼ teaspoon fine sea salt
1½ cups (188 grams) all-purpose flour
A pinch of sea salt flakes, like Maldon, if using (see headnote)

Preheat the oven to 350 degrees, and butter and flour a 9-inch fluted tart pan with a removable bottom.

Spread the sliced almonds in a single layer on a baking sheet and toast them in the preheated oven for 5 to 7 minutes, until fragrant. They should color only lightly.

Whisk together the melted butter and 1½ cups sugar in a large bowl. Add one egg, whisk until fully incorporated, then add the other and whisk some more. Add the almond extract, vanilla, and salt, and whisk well, until smooth. With a rubber spatula, fold in the flour until just combined.

Spread the batter evenly in the prepared pan and scatter the toasted almonds, sea salt flakes, if using, and 1 tablespoon sugar over top. Bake for 35 minutes, until the cake peeking through the almonds takes on a faintly rosy color (this cake blushes more than it browns), and a tester inserted into the center comes out clean. Cool on a rack until nearly room temperature, then ease the cake out of the pan and cool the rest of the way.

Serves 8 to 10.

CHAPTER 3

Passing Through

At first, I didn't understand what all the fuss was about. I was in the ICU. The Pit. Okay. But the scans had shown nothing broken in my brain, and this sounded like good news to me. A doctor stopped by my corner of the Pit and basically confirmed as much. He said that sometimes, for unknown reasons, there is a spontaneous bleed, and then the brain just heals itself up.

I liked how he called it "a bleed." As a noun the word was far less forbidding, like how smoking can kill you but going for "a smoke" sounds all right. A bleed was no big deal. A dot of blood from a finger prick, a scraped knee. He said I'd be out of there in a few days.

Meanwhile, I lay in bed feeling not bad at all. The nurses brought me foam lollypops dunked in water for me to swipe around my mouth, since I wasn't yet allowed to drink. The first one was a revelation, but I was over it by the fourth or fifth, and getting thirsty. So that wasn't great. Mostly, though, I felt okay—and vaguely guilty about that, like when you're home sick as a kid and the Tylenol kicks in, and you suddenly feel quite well, but get to go on watching *The Price Is Right* and eating all the Jell-O you want.

Everything had taken on a sheen of novelty—the monitors, the buttons that adjusted my bed. When you turn eight in my family, you get to go on a trip somewhere by yourself with the grandparents. They took me to Toronto. It was only Canada, but it was still a foreign country, the first I'd ever visited. I adored the marks of foreignness: the highway signs in French, the kilometers per hour, the colorful money, the black squirrels. I liked the feeling of heightened curiosity that came with being somewhere new. Living amid the unfamiliar made me feel up for anything.

The hospital had a similar effect, at first. I'd seen a lot of these things in the movies or on TV, but never up close. Electrodes stuck to my chest measured my heart rate. A glowing red meter taped to my index finger checked the oxygen in my blood. (My "E.T. finger," Eli called it.) A catheter emptied my bladder into a baggie at the foot of the bed. An IV machine hooked up to my right arm would beep when the liquid neared empty, and often for no reason at all.

While I wasn't exactly comfortable with all those tubes and wires poking into my body, it was too soon for them to be anything more than a nuisance. Meanwhile, it was all so interesting. I'd hold my breath to see if I could get the numbers on the screens to jump around. I'd lift an arm and watch the lines on the EKG spike. It wasn't the end of the world to be stuck here for a few days. I was just passing through, a tourist on my way home.

My family started arriving early that evening. Eli's parents drove from New Jersey and got there first. I'd been keeping myself occupied by translating songs into Yiddish in my head, and I was in the middle of "Over the Rainbow" (*ergets, ibern regnboygn*) when they arrived. I asked my mother-in-law, Sarah, a native Yiddish speaker, if she knew of a specific word for "chimney tops." "Rest," she said and patted my arm.

I *was* resting. This was the longest I'd done nothing in years. The previous semester, in addition to studying for my exams, I'd finished up my coursework, taught two classes, organized a conference with a colleague, and written a paper that I'd presented there. No wonder my brain had sprung a leak.

My father showed up next. I was feeling so well that I was just plain old happy to see him. "I'm okay, Dad," I said. "Really, I'm fine. Could you tell him?" I asked the nurse.

Finally, my mother arrived. She'd gotten a call from Adena first thing that morning. When she hung up the phone, she grabbed a few things, got in the car, and drove. It's almost eleven hours by car from Orange Village, Ohio, to Burlington, Vermont, but this didn't surprise me. Her response to potential crisis is locomotion. When she arrived, she looked awake, alert, and beautiful—especially so, even—as though she'd been staying at an inn around the corner, heard I was laid up, then showered, dressed, and walked the two blocks over. I remember her by the entranceway of the Pit, scanning for me while the nurse pointed. I hoped hard she wouldn't cry. When she didn't, it seemed a great act of kindness.

After my parents had come and gone, my overnight nurse appeared. She was petite and pretty with blond hair to her chin. Like everyone I'd met that day, she put me right at ease. She told me that since nothing had come up on my scans, it was now official that I wouldn't be having surgery, and I could put something in my stomach.

I began with a sip of water. I couldn't believe its softness, a silk ribbon tumbling down my throat. I could have a lemon ice, she offered, and when it came, I smiled in recognition. It was a brand called

Luigi's, the same kind that my in-laws stock in their freezer. Eli and his siblings prefer the strawberry, which is sweeter, and softer against the spoon. I say there's nothing like lemon after a Friday night meal of meat, more meat, and potatoes, and my father-in-law, Steve, agrees. He stomps up the steps from the basement freezer, calling, "Luigi's! Luigi's!" in a fake Italian accent, hands over the strawberry cups to the others with equally phony disdain, and sits down next to me with the lemons. The others empty their cups first, and we're left scraping away together, just us two. That I had a lemon Luigi's in my hand that first night in the ICU felt like a very good sign.

When I finished eating, the nurse suggested I sleep. She said that, if I wanted, she could rub my back for a while. She helped me roll onto my side, slathered her hands with lotion, and stroked downward between my shoulder blades. Her hands were cool. I relaxed. Exhaustion tugged at my eyelids. I felt so comfortable there, so taken care of, with my family tucked into motel beds down the road. The pain was gone. There would be no surgery. That there was still blood of unknown origins pooling in my brain didn't faze me.

But my nurse that night, she knew. She must have. She knew what happens when the body tries to reabsorb blood that's where it never should have been. As she smoothed the lotion over my body, I let myself sink into sleep. I looked forward to waking up the next morning. I looked forward to going home.

CHAPTER 4

At the Table

Eli and I met at the table. It was the first Friday night of my first week of my freshman year of college in New York City, and I had walked the three blocks from my dormitory to sit in the common room of another dormitory and eat a proper family-style meal. Yes, you read that correctly. I was eighteen years old with my parents five hundred miles away, the entire city at my fingertips, a loaded MetroCard that my grandparents had given me for graduation, and, TGIF, I was going to spend my evening in the faintly damp-smelling common room of a college dormitory eating chicken.

The invitation was for a traditional Jewish Friday night dinner, the first of many student-hosted Sabbath meals I'd attend over the years. The table that night was actually several tables, dragged from neighboring suites and pushed together into a long banquet-style strip by the wall and covered in overlapping paper tablecloths. There were a lot of us, sixteen at least. We had to squeeze to fit around the table, and those of us on the wall side had to inch our way to our seats, single file. Across from me was a skinny boy who'd brushed out his curls into a wavy, sideways flop.

It was Eli, of course. He was totally annoying.

He sat all crooked with his left arm draped over the back of his chair, and when he spoke, which was often, he'd cock his head to the side and hold out his right hand, palm up, as if expecting a tip. He wasn't loud or rude, in fact, he seemed smart, but he was talking about the gap year he'd just completed in Israel, and all he could do was complain. Let me rephrase that: His parents had just paid for him to live for an entire year overseas, and all he could do was complain.

Eli grew up in an Orthodox Jewish community where the norm is to spend a year after high school in Jerusalem at a yeshiva, a religious academy for the study of Jewish law. Eli's parents are educated, left-leaning intellectuals. His father, Steve, is a psychiatrist who adores German opera and studies Hegel and Kant for fun. His mother, Sarah, is a social worker who once chained herself to an embassy in the name of human rights. The Orthodox Jewish schools that Eli attended as a kid were fairly liberal. Somehow, though, he ended up in a yeshiva in Israel that was not. According to the rabbis there, university could lead only to sin and blasphemy. They urged him to give up secular pursuits, spend his days studying Talmud and little else. Eli resisted, to say the least.

He skipped class. He found a bookstore that sold Penguin Classics, those paperbacks with the yellow covers, for just ten shekels each—no more than two or three American dollars—and picked up one after another. He read *The Iliad*, *The Odyssey*, *The Secret Garden*, the Foundation series by Isaac Asimov. Daniel DeFoe, Dickens, Jules Verne, Proust. Any English-language anything he could get his hands on over there. He made it through the year that way.

I didn't know any of this that night at the table. All I saw was a thankless kid, rocking back and forth on the hind legs of his chair. We didn't exchange a single word that night. Sometimes, in the dining hall or around campus, I'd pass him, just a chest and a head floating above the giant black portfolio he carried around for his drawing class and two legs sticking out below. We never waved hello.

The following fall, he joined the choir that I'd been singing with all freshman year. He had come into the audition with a yellow Discman, stuck one headphone into his ear to find his starting note, and, looking very serious indeed, busted out a colossally earnest rendition of "Brian Wilson" by the Barenaked Ladies. He had never sung in a choir before.

Between us, he was just okay. But we'd lost a tenor to graduation, and Eli had potential.

"He's a cutie," my friend Robin said after he left the room. I shrugged and said he wasn't my type. (As though I had one. I was dating my first-ever boyfriend at the time, the same guy who'd been my first kiss at age eighteen and a half, less than a year before.) More to the point, everyone agreed that Eli seemed like a good guy, which, when you're a group of only sixteen singers with away gigs most weekends, is important. Eli was in. And after a few rehearsals even I had to admit he was kind of likable.

For one thing, he brought the best snacks. Sunflower seeds, salted, still in their shells, pints of fresh berries, sugar snap peas, dried cherries. These things are expensive, splurges on a college budget, but he shared. I'd never even seen a dried cherry before, nor had I ever been particularly moved one way or the other by a dried fruit. Dried cherries, though! Intense like you'd never expect from something so shriveled and small. A single cherry could launch its sweet-tart flavor straight up into your soft palate. Wake your salivary glands right up.

Eli was taking a sculpture class that semester and would often come to rehearsal straight from the studio with smudges on his white tee and his chin-length curls pulled back into a ponytail. It surprises me how much I remember about him from the early days of our friendship: his stride, how he was always leaning back slightly, even while walking, his skinny silhouette, his hands crammed into the pockets of his wool coat. "Hey, Jess, howya doin'?" he'd say. I liked that.

The following semester, I enrolled in a basic drawing class. I didn't know the first thing about sketching pencils, charcoals, or vinyl erasers, so I asked Eli, the only visual arts major I knew, to accompany me down to Pearl Paint on Canal. We'd never hung out just the two of us. It's a long subway ride from 116th to Canal Street and back, and we talked the whole way.

I told him about how coming to school in New York had felt like coming home, even though I'd moved away from the city when I was five, about these classes called "ear training" that I had to take as part of my music major to learn how to transcribe music the way you would a spoken dictation, and how I wasn't very good at it. He told me about his own drawing classes, what made his instructor so good, his frustrations when he put pencil to paper. His second major was computer science, and he talked about coding in terms I'd never considered. It was a form of art, too, he said, a way of bringing something beautiful into the world that hadn't been there before. Eli knew stuff about buildings and architecture and the history of squatters' rights. In fact, he seemed to know something about everything. He didn't lecture or flaunt. Rather, it was as though his whole life he'd been quietly gathering treasures. Little nuggets and gems of things he had heard or seen or read, and he was just uncurling his fingers to share them.

I want to pause here to cross my heart and swear that the thought of Eli Schleifer as love interest never entered my mind. Not once. Yes, he was easy to be around, and he made me laugh, and think, and taught me new things all the time. Whenever we spoke, my skin felt more like my own. But, you know, that's all.

Besides, he had a girlfriend. A smart, sexy, funny, gorgeous girlfriend named Rebecca, someone he'd agonized over for months until they'd finally gotten together and who, in my estimation, was his perfect match. Then there was the matter of my own sweet, handsome boyfriend. Which wasn't a "matter" at all except, perhaps, for the fact that I was secretly having to convince myself to love this very good man.

People sometimes ask me if there were signs—a faint hum of attraction, a "what if?" moment in the privacy of my mind—and if, looking back, I can see them. Nope. Sometimes it takes time to know what you know.

Eli's Oatmeal Cookies

Eli doesn't like sweets—nobody's perfect—but he does have a soft spot for a few select things, oatmeal cookies being one of them. These are his favorite. They're big, chewy saucers, crisp around the edges, with just enough whole wheat flour to warm up the flavor. To scoop the dough for these, I use a 1½-tablespoon cookie scoop, piling two level scoops, one on top of the other.

   1½ cups (135 grams) rolled oats (not instant)
   1 cup (125 grams) all-purpose flour
   ½ cup (57 grams) whole wheat flour
   ½ teaspoon baking soda
   ½ teaspoon baking powder
   ½ teaspoon cinnamon
   1 cup (2 sticks; 226 grams) unsalted butter, melted
   ½ cup (100 grams) dark brown sugar
   ½ cup (100 grams) granulated sugar

1 teaspoon fine-grain salt

1 large egg

1 teaspoon pure vanilla extract

Mix the first six ingredients (the oats through the cinnamon) in a medium bowl. Combine the melted butter, the sugars, and salt in a large bowl and whisk well. Then add the egg and vanilla and whisk until smooth. Add the dry ingredients to the butter mixture and stir with a rubber spatula or wooden spoon until just combined. Do not overmix. Cover the bowl and refrigerate for 20 to 30 minutes, until the dough is cool and firm but still scoopable.

While the dough is resting, heat the oven to 325 degrees and line a baking sheet with parchment paper. Using 3 level tablespoons per cookie, scoop the dough onto the prepared baking sheet. The cookies will spread as they bake, so leave 2 to 3 inches between each mound of dough. I fit 8 cookies, staggered, per pan.

Bake for 18 to 22 minutes until golden brown. Slide the parchment paper with the cookies onto a rack and cool completely. Repeat with the remaining dough, making sure to begin with a room temperature baking sheet.

Makes about 16 cookies.

CHAPTER 5

Patient

I don't remember the start of the pain. All I know is, I was in it, sunk.

I felt around for the shape of it. A headache has texture and fault lines. You can rotate your neck and sometimes find them, bury your face in a pillow, dig your finger into your temple, hard. You may not get relief, but you can at least make contact, push the pain around a bit, and there's comfort in that.

This pain was different. Liquid cement and formless, everywhere, with no place to grab on to. I couldn't move.

When you bang your hip on the nightstand, your body knows what to do. We're designed to get hurt, to bruise, and then to reabsorb the spilled blood beneath the surface of our skin. Something else happens when the blood is in your brain. We're not designed for that. You typically do not recover from a bleeding brain, so there's no efficient biological system in place for healing, nowhere for the blood to go as long as it's trapped up there in your skull. And so it travels down along your spinal column looking for a way out, or a way back in. The pain of that seepage, that slow crawl, is an ocean. If the medications touched it, I couldn't tell.

Suddenly, the machines that I'd treated like toys seemed to have something to do with me. My condition was no graver now that I was in pain. My body was suffering from the aftermath of the hemorrhage that had already occurred, not under a new attack. But the pain turned me into a patient.

A few minutes went by, or hours, or days. People came. They must have, though I couldn't tell. Pain like this is the ultimate privacy. And then it was gone. I didn't come out of it in the way you sometimes feel yourself waking up, conscious before you've opened your eyes. I was just in my bed again, alone, with the feeling that something terrible had left the room.

Patty, the nurse who'd welcomed me to the Pit, was back on duty. I was relieved not to have to meet someone new, and it took me by surprise how happy I was to see her. I'd been there only forty-eight hours, but I already knew she was my favorite. It felt good to have a favorite, to have some kind of preference in that place.

That night, I heard groaning coming from somewhere in the Pit. Actually, it was more of a loud gurgle, like a groan that had been shoved under water against its will. It went on for hours. The voice belonged to a man, someone older. He was across the way from me and over to the right. He sounded frantic, as though he were trying to lift something too heavy off his own body. I wondered if he was in pain like the pain I'd been in the night before.

When a nurse came to change my IV bag, I asked if he was okay, and she said not to worry. By then he was shouting. She told me his name, which I'm not even sure she was allowed to do: Marshall.

I awoke the next morning in motion, on my way down to an MRI. Someone was pushing my bed from behind. I'd already had an angiogram, a procedure where they thread a tiny catheter up through your groin, shoot your brain full of dye, and take pictures. They hadn't found anything broken, but the images had been so clouded by the spilled blood in my brain that they wanted to check again. To be safe. They couldn't do an angiogram this time because the blood vessels in my head were in spasm. That's common after a hemorrhage and makes the risk of stroke during an angiogram too high. MRI is a noninvasive technique. They hoped it might show something new.

I didn't mind the narrowness of the tube, the cage that came down over my face, or the clicking and buzzing in there. The technician told me it was very important that I keep as still as possible, and I was glad to have something to focus on. After a few minutes, though, the hard scanner bed started digging into the back of my skull. Just one angry spot, at first, right above the base of my neck. *There must be a peg or something sticking up there*, I thought. I could feel it drilling into my head. When they were done I'd sit up, I figured, and the pain would stop. *Don't move. It can't be long.* But by the time they were sliding me out of the machine I knew there was no peg. The pain, the big liquid one, was coming back.

A new nurse appeared to return me to the ICU. She punched her fist in the air as she told me it was time to go, and said, "Cool beans!" She pushed the bed in an exaggerated way, bent at the waist and elbows, as though she were acting the whole thing out. The way she moved reminded me of a high school cheerleader, electrically upbeat, not entirely comfortable in her body, but faking it as best she could. "Cool beans!" she said a couple more times on the way, filling the silence.

A room had opened up in the ICU, an actual room with a window on one side and a wall made of glass that looked out onto the nurses' station when the curtains weren't drawn. My parents were there waiting for me. I tried to tell them that something bad was happening again, but no one seemed to understand what I was saying. My father asked the nurse to page the doctor. He looked scared. "Okay," she said, "cool beans!" as she slipped out the door.

The pain was metallic and one thousand pounds. I was alone in it, again.

Someone was in the chair beside my bed. Eli. He reached over me and balanced a fresh ice pack on my head, wedged it into place with an extra pillow. I needed his face to look like his face, but instead it looked hard and flat, strange in a way I couldn't figure out, as though someone had found the knobs that control brightness and contrast and turned them way down. It was the kind of face you wear when something has happened, something that annoys you or hurts you, but you don't want to say what it is.

This face was new. I'd never seen it, because when there was something to say, we'd always say. That was what had kept us going the first two years we were dating, and I say "dating" only because I'm not aware of a word that means "newly in love and living continents apart." We spent our first year "together" with me in England working on a master's degree, and Eli in Seattle, where he'd taken a job after college. The following year, I moved to Jerusalem and he stayed put, halfway around the globe. We met up two or three times a year in his country, or mine, or somewhere in-between. On our way to the airport at the end of one of these visits, we passed a store called Blinds to Go. I started it:

"Blinds to Go? How else would you take your blinds?"

"What?"

"Who buys blinds 'to stay'?"

Eli jumped right in. "The venetian, please. To go!"

"On second thought," I added, "I think I'll bring my windows in and enjoy those blinds right here."

We were champs at running commentary. A brain hemorrhage, then, and its attending drama? Surely we had something to say about that. "Are you okay?" I kept asking. "Are we okay," as though the crisis here were marital, a misunderstanding the two of us could work out. For the first time since I'd known him, Eli barely spoke.

I wanted to sit up in bed, grab him by the shoulders, shake him, hug him, shout, "Hey!" and bury my face in his neck. I wanted to step outside of all this, the real me with the real Eli, and talk about what had happened. I'd ask about all the parts I couldn't quite remember, and what the doctors had said so far. I'd ask him what I looked like when the pain and morphine carried me off, how much time was really passing between one fully conscious moment and the next. He'd tell me what he was thinking when he was sitting by my bed, and what he was up to in the world outside. Where was he staying? With whom? Where was he when he got the call? And then what happened? And then what?

"Are my parents behaving themselves?" I'd want to know.

"Sort of," he'd say with a laugh, and I'd make him tell me everything.

Eli sometimes does this thing when he's sharing a story, where he'll come to the end and insist that's all he's got. Never believe him. There's always more to it at the very edges of his memory. You just have to know the right questions to ask, the right buttons to push, and that's what I'd do here, until he'd laid the whole thing out and we'd made sense of it, together.

The MRI had been inconclusive. I'd need another angiogram after all. An ultrasound was scheduled to see if my vessels had calmed down enough, and I asked my parents, both of them, to come with me. They walked on either side of my bed as the nurse wheeled me through the halls. The last time I'd been with both of them together was at my wedding less than three years earlier, one of them on each side, escorting me down the aisle. It was too narrow for three, so I'd had to hold them close, looped under opposite arms, in a not-quite family hug.

The technician squirted gel onto my face and neck and started moving the wand around. My parents were looking at each other, exchanging glances the way they had when they were married and I was a child. It was the kind of thing I'd felt back then but registered only when it was gone: that for a child there is shelter in the everyday words and glances shared by the grown-ups in the room.

I'd have an angiogram the next day. I was glad. Information was the only momentum I had, and I liked knowing that there would be more of it, soon.

The lights were dim when I saw the four of them looking down at me: Eli, his father, mine, and someone I'd already met, but couldn't place. The doctors had been hard to keep track of—residents, fellows rotating in and out and around my bed. I hadn't picked up that the doctor standing there now was the one in charge: Dr. Bruce Tranmer, a brain surgeon. No one was smiling.

My family appeared composed in the way someone cinched into a girdle appears thin: stiff, unbreathing, erect. Eli's father was flushed and mine looked gray. Eli's face had flattened out again into a solid wall, and I was suddenly sure that the angiogram had turned up evidence that soon I would be dead. It was the only explanation for the way they were looking at me. I sucked in my breath and grew still, bracing myself for the news.

Eli spoke first. "Jess, they found an aneurysm in your brain. You're going to need surgery to repair it."

An aneurysm. A tiny, misshapen estuary where blood had pooled along the weakened wall of a vessel until, one morning on a treadmill, it popped. Dr. Tranmer explained that there are two different kinds. The first is called a berry aneurysm. It's round, like a berry, ballooning outward from the blood vessel through a thin "stem." With a berry aneurysm, you can sometimes avoid open-brain surgery and instead fill it with platinum coils. The surgeon snakes a catheter through your groin up into your brain and places the coils through it from outside your body. The other kind, a fusiform aneurysm, is shaped more like a bean. It lies lower and flatter against the vessel and connects along its entire length. Without a stem to keep the coils from just falling out, fusiform aneurysms need to be clipped. And the only way to do that is to cut open your head. I had this second kind.

"But you can fix it?" I asked. I wasn't sure I understood. Dr. Tranmer nodded. "Yes."

The plan was to saw through my skull, slice into my brain, and seal off the aneurysm with a titanium clip the shape of a tiny clothespin. Dr. Tranmer dropped one into my hand for me to inspect. He'd place the clip along the base of the aneurysm, he explained, cutting off its blood flow. The aneurysm would wither—I pictured a flattened bubble on a sheet of Bubble Wrap—and the vessel would heal beneath the strengthened wall formed by the length of the clip.

Now, when you are certain that you have but a few last gasps on this earth, and someone tells you that, actually, the news is brain surgery, the world looks suddenly rosy. What I felt, above all, was relief. Also a relief was the fact that I was back to feeling quite well. There was no more pain. In its place, euphoria had landed. I could sit up in bed now. Roll over. Listen to episode after episode of *This*

American Life. Just being able to eat again made the hospital meals a treat, the way airplane food feels special by virtue of the fact that you eat it thirty thousand feet in the air.

Even the nights weren't particularly unpleasant. They were long, though, and came with heparin shots in my belly that weirded me out. A shot in the belly seemed different from a shot in the arm or the hip or the butt, places better fashioned to accept such an affront. A belly is defenseless and lovely. I dreaded watching the needles sink down into mine.

Every morning was the same. One of Dr. Tranmer's residents, Dr. Link, would come by and hold out his fingers for me to squeeze. At some point I stopped waiting for the string of questions and answered them unprompted: "Two thousand eight." "George Bush." "Burlington, Vermont." Or sometimes, if I was feeling fancy, *"Fletcher Allen hospital* in Burlington, Vermont." He said the same thing every single day before he left: "Hang in there." Dr. Link was handsome in a strapping, Clark Kent kind of way and I started to think of those words as his scripted line. I told the nurses, and one morning as he was finishing up they gathered just outside my room. "Hang in there," he said, and they giggled.

One of my professors called, the one who was supposed to examine me in Russian history a few weeks later. I felt nervous telling him that I would perhaps need to postpone the exam and was surprised when he laughed and told me that the department administrator had already completed the paperwork for my medical leave that semester. *An entire semester?* That seemed excessive. I felt great. So great, that I half expected Dr. Tranmer to appear with the news that the brain surgery he'd mentioned wouldn't be necessary after all.

A few days into my hospital stay, my father had given me a small stuffed bear with an orange ribbon tied around its neck. I named him Marshall after the man from the Pit. I couldn't stop thinking about him. He'd sounded so sick, and I'd heard that he'd had no visitors. Meanwhile, there I was with an entire crew; a stuffed bear; piles of cards; a windowsill crammed with chocolates; a drawing pad and bucket of markers that my mother had brought me; and a stuffed, smiley-faced flower with bright pink petals that, frankly, in the gauzy light of the ICU, gave me the creeps. I kept thinking of myself in relation to Marshall: his aloneness, his grave illness, versus my doting family and soon-to-be perfect health. I pictured poor Marshall languishing in the Pit while I resumed my life at home, far away from here. This was the way I'd positioned us in my mind, his well-being and mine on opposite sides of a wheel, locked in an inverse position.

The next day, I asked how he was doing. He'd gone home.

CHAPTER 6

Z-i-t-i

Long before I loved Eli Schleifer, I loved the way he ate. He always seemed to eat so well, at least by college student standards. Those rehearsal snacks were only the beginning. Most of us made do with the complimentary slice of tomato they would add to your bagel at the campus café. Eli liked lox on his, so he got lox. And he bought grapes. Never mind their steep price per pound. Frozen, he'll tell you, they make the best dessert. ("Almost as good as *unfrozen* grapes," our friend Eitan likes to say.)

Eli wasn't buying steak dinners or fine wines. Just little luxuries here and there—fresh-squeezed orange juice, for example—that don't normally fit into a college budget. He paid most of his own way through college, so it's not as if he had tons of money lying around. Whatever he did have, he was happy to spend on food. Getting to eat what he wanted to eat was worth it.

"Why food?" I once asked him. "Why not buy, I don't know, nicer shoes?"

Eli shrugged. "I was hungry."

Our sophomore year of college, a semester after he joined our choir, we took a social history class together. We sat directly across the seminar table from each other, closest to the instructor on either side, and at the break, together with most of our class, we would go to the student-run kosher deli across the hall. I'd never been a fan of deli sandwiches. Too salty, too flabby. The mustard was the best part. I'd usually get a knish, instead. (Though, admittedly, the mustard was the best part there, too.)

Eli did not approve. So one day, he ordered for me. Heat the corned beef, he told the student behind the counter, and stuff some coleslaw in there. Coleslaw. Right *on the sandwich*. Warmed through, the corned beef's fat didn't squeak or ball up on my tongue. The meat was juicy now, tender and soft. And the coleslaw. There was crunch! This was deli reborn.

A hot corned beef sandwich with coleslaw became my regular order, and when I asked Eli to eat his sandwich slowly, please, so that I wouldn't be the last one chewing and wiping my lips back in class, he laughed and said okay.

Meanwhile, Eli was expanding his own culinary frontiers. He'd grown up observing kashrut, the Jewish dietary laws. Some foods, like pork and shellfish, were entirely off-limits, and his family had separate sets of dishes for meat and dairy foods, which must be eaten apart. We did, too, growing up, though my mother did it mostly out of respect for her own parents, and because it was what she had always known. Eli's family went further. Even outside their home they ate only food that was certified kosher, cooked in kosher ovens in kosher pans, and served on kosher plates. Vacations meant lugging coolers filled with tuna sandwiches and hard-boiled eggs. They always stayed in rental apartments with kitchens, his mother unpacking her own pots, foil roasting tins, even a food processor, while they all settled in. When I met Eli, he'd never eaten so much as a dinner roll from a restaurant that wasn't kosher.

All of which is to explain the following scene. I was walking along Broadway one night, on my way back to the dorm, when I ran into Eli with a couple of crumpled napkins in his hand. He was flushed and grinning.

"I just ate my first nonkosher food," he announced in a half whisper. He looked spooked.

"What was it?" I wanted to know, imagining a cheeseburger, or a hot dog from a stand.

"Pizza."

"With pepperoni? Sausage?"

"Cheese."

A slice of *cheese pizza*. This was the giant leap from the strictures of his youth.

Eli had never been what you might call "a believer." But when you're a kid, what feels normal and right is whatever you know, so he'd always walked the walk, abstaining from electricity, writing, and driving on the Sabbath; blessing his food; wearing a yarmulke on his head and symbolic fringes under his shirt. This was his world. His family and friends did all these things, too. Stepping back was anything but natural. Each transgression had to be a conscious, deliberate act. He forced himself to turn on the lights and listen to music on Saturday afternoons. He ate more pizza. By the end of the year, he was leaving his yarmulke at home.

The complicating thing, here, is that even as Eli wanted out, there was much that he loved to keep him, especially around the table: the traditional songs after Friday night meals, playing board games with his brothers on long Saturday afternoons, unplugged from the world in accordance with the Sabbath laws. He loved decorating the sukkah, a backyard hut, for the harvest holiday of Sukkot every fall, rolling out the bamboo mat for the roof and covering it with leaves, hanging the foil peacock that hung over his father's chair and the illustrated mats for the walls. They ate seven nights of meals out there, the laughter and singing from neighbors' sukkot audible over their own.

Eli wasn't about to let go of these things. He may not have wanted to feel bound by that world, but he wanted very much still to be in it. So, even as his own religious practice waned, he lived year after year with his Orthodox Jewish friends. This way, he was "grandfathered in," he once told me, included despite whatever he now believed. He liked that.

When we weren't traveling on weekends with our choir, Eli would often host Friday night dinners. Most student-hosted dinners were potluck, like the one where we first met, with upwards of ten people crowded around too-small tables or sitting on made-up beds. Eli would cap his guest list at six and make all the food himself. Most of his recipes were Schleifer family classics: chicken coated in his mother's preferred brand of Russian dressing, tossed with bread crumbs in a Ziploc bag, transferred to a pan, and baked. This was "chicken in a bag," something he'd made as a kid when his parents worked late. Also in this category: tuna casserole and baked ziti, which the Schleifers pronounce "zitty," as though the pasta were seventeen and in need of a deep-cleansing face mask.

"Zitty, zee-tee, what did I know from Italian?" my mother-in-law explained. Sarah is the child of two Polish immigrants who spoke only Yiddish at home. Salt and pepper, she says, were the only "spices" she ever saw in her mother's kitchen. She learned to cook from cookbooks and found the baked ziti recipe when Eli and his three siblings were small. Z-i-t-i: She'd never seen this word before. But baked pasta bubbling with tomato sauce and cheese? As Sarah would say, what could be wrong with that?

Eli made new things, too. A salad of spinach, mushrooms, strawberries, and candied pecans. Chicken breasts stuffed with apricots and greens. He had a juicer and would shake up too-sweet cocktails of fresh apple juice and Midori that we all thought were terrific. He didn't do soups or hot beverages, period, which might have troubled me if I didn't find the particularity of it so endearing. This was a man who knew his own preferences and tastes and honored them. Politely refusing the soft-serve strawberry ice cream at the register because, if you recall, he ordered the strawberry hard-scoop, wasn't fussiness for its own sake, but deliberate living. I liked this guy more than I knew.

Saucy Baked Ziti

Don't tell my mother-in-law, or for that matter my husband, but for a long time I just didn't get baked ziti. It seemed like the no-man's-land of pasta dishes, lying somewhere between pasta with sauce and lasagna, and less delicious than both. This ziti changed my mind. It is its own terrific thing, saucy and full flavored with a bit of heat. (If you're not into spicy, reduce the crushed red pepper in the tomato sauce by half a teaspoon or so.) I like the crisp bread-crumb topping and the hint of nutmeg, which may sound like a strange addition, but you'll be glad it's there. Don't let the béchamel sauce intimidate you. Just be sure to warm the milk and add it slowly to the pot to keep the sauce from breaking.

Despite the name of this recipe, Eli and I have discovered that we like it best with rigatoni, another tubelike pasta that's larger than ziti and ridged along the surface. Oh, and use the best canned tomatoes you can find for this dish, which, of course, is a matter of taste. I like Muir Glen.

This recipe is adapted from one that chef Mario Batali shared with Dana Cowin for her book *Mastering My Mistakes in the Kitchen*. It's great at the center of a casual dinner party, with a big salad, a bowl of olives, and a couple bottles of wine.

For the tomato sauce:

>4 tablespoons olive oil
>
>3 garlic cloves, minced
>
>1 teaspoon crushed red pepper, plus more to taste
>
>2 28-ounce cans whole peeled tomatoes
>
>1 teaspoon fine sea salt, plus more to taste

For the béchamel:

>2 tablespoons unsalted butter
>
>2 tablespoons all-purpose flour
>
>2 cups whole milk, warmed (but not boiled)
>
>½ teaspoon fine sea salt, plus more to taste
>
>¼ teaspoon nutmeg, plus more to taste

For the rest of the dish:

>1 pound dry ziti or rigatoni
>
>8 ounces fresh mozzarella cheese, cut into ½-inch cubes
>
>1 cup (50 grams) freshly grated Parmesan
>
>1 cup (50 grams) panko bread crumbs
>
>A pinch or two of nutmeg
>
>½ teaspoon crushed red pepper (optional)
>
>2 tablespoons olive oil
>
>A handful of fresh basil leaves, sliced or torn into small pieces

Position a rack in the top third of the oven, and preheat to 375 degrees. Brush a 9-by-13-inch ceramic or glass baking dish with olive oil.

Make the tomato sauce:

Pour the 4 tablespoons olive oil into a 3- or 4-quart saucepan and warm over medium-high heat until it shimmers. Stir in the garlic and crushed red pepper and cook for a minute or so, until fragrant. Add the tomatoes, smooshing them up with your hands as you drop them into the pot. Dump in any juices left in the cans, stir in the salt, turn the heat up to high, and bring to a boil. Lower the heat and simmer, stirring occasionally, for about 10 minutes, until the sauce thickens slightly. Taste, and add more salt and crushed red pepper, if you'd like. Remove the pot from the heat and set aside.

Meanwhile, make the béchamel:

Melt the butter in a 3- or 4-quart saucepan over medium heat. Add the flour and stir for a couple of minutes, to form a pale brown paste. Very slowly pour in the warm milk while whisking continuously. Bring the sauce to a boil and cook for about 5 minutes, stirring the whole time, until it thickens. Remove the pot from the heat, stir in the salt and nutmeg, and taste. If you prefer more salt or nutmeg, stir it in, and set the sauce aside.

Make the pasta and assemble the dish:

Bring a large pot of water to a boil and toss in a few hefty pinches of salt. Add the pasta, and cook until it's 3 or 4 minutes short of done. (It will cook the rest of the way through in the oven.) Drain the pasta and transfer it to your largest bowl.

Add the tomato sauce, béchamel, mozzarella, and about three-quarters of the Parmesan to the ziti and mix well. Transfer the mixture to the prepared baking dish and scatter the rest of the Parmesan over top. In a small bowl, toss the bread crumbs with a nice pinch of nutmeg, plus another ½ teaspoon or so of crushed red pepper if you want some extra heat, mix with the 2 tablespoons olive oil, and sprinkle over the ziti.

Bake until the ziti is bubbling and the top is brown, about 15 minutes. Remove from the oven and let rest for 10 minutes, then scatter the sliced basil over the top and serve.

Serves 6 to 8.

CHAPTER 7

The Moon Out of the Sky

When I visit someplace new, my favorite thing to do is eat. And walk—preferably to a place where I can eat some more. Florence is for art, yes. The Uffizi. The Pitti Palace. The Galleria dell'Accademia. But I'd have waited in lines twice as long for the tiny strawberries that Eli and I found at the outdoor market there, for the way they dissolved in our mouths like sucking candies and turned our fingertips pink.

Food is more than what we put into our bodies when we are wherever we are. It's the feel of a place, something language can't get at, the memory of a place as it forms. Montreal is a loaf of bread sticky with dates, hazelnuts tucked into its crumb. It's the crackle of crust as we ripped into it with our hands. Jerusalem is the fruit stall at the end of the block, persimmons and pomegranates in heaps, pomelos the size of my head. Wherever I am, food is what makes me feel there.

Even when "there" is an ICU hospital bed in Burlington, Vermont. Never mind that it's the city where a surgeon unpacked my brain on an operating table. That I was doing very little eating and even less walking didn't matter, since I had a devoted squad of visitors committed to both of these things.

My family had more or less moved to Burlington during the early weeks of my illness, staying in hotels, inns, and, in my mother's case, a guest room at a nearby convent. ICU visiting hours are limited, on again, off again, throughout the day. I'd watch the clock and wait, imagining my people at restaurant tables, in line for coffee, choosing bananas from produce displays. When they'd finally file into my room, I'd make them tell me all about it.

Which is how, having only ever passed through the city in the back of an ambulance, I became deeply acquainted with where the people of Burlington go to eat. There's a café called Mirabelles, where my mother tried steel-cut oatmeal for the first, second, third, and fourth times, in rapid succession. She reported on each encounter, and though I knew firsthand the extra chew and heft of steel-cut oats, how they stand up to a long, slow simmer and transform into a creamy pudding, I looked forward to each retelling. My brother-in-law liked the vegan French toast at the Magnolia Bistro, and though my aggressively nonvegan husband must have gone there just to humor him, he liked it, too. There were the chocolate chip cookies baked at the inn where my stepmother, Amy, stayed for a few nights, and the health food store where my father would buy me flavored soda waters and line them up on the ledge by my window. People brought me menus from everywhere. I studied them. It felt good just knowing what was out there. And even better when I finally got to taste it.

Eli had driven his road bike up from Cambridge to ride between hospital visits. He was training for a century ride, one hundred miles through the five boroughs of New York City. The event was still a few weeks out, and we agreed that he should carry on with his training. I'd be postsurgery by the time the ride came around. I wanted him to do it.

So, while I lay in bed staring at the whiteboard where the nurses wrote the date each day, he rode. I liked to picture him flying down the country roads. The padded shorts that endowed his narrow frame with a butt, the yellow and black jersey zipped up to his chin, sunglasses wrapped around his head. He looked like a wasp with knees.

On one of his rides, Eli passed a sign for pick-your-own berries. When he got back to town, he announced to my family that he was going to get some for me, and would anyone like to join him? And so it was that Eli, my in-laws, and my divorced parents squeezed into a single car, bumped down a dirt road, and rolled to a stop alongside a mosquito-infested orchard.

It had rained recently, and my mother was concerned about the mud. My mother-in-law was concerned about the thorns. They were all concerned about the mosquitoes. But these people would gladly have shot the moon out of the sky for me that day. As it turned out, they did something even better: venturing into the raspberry patch, slapping at their arms and the backs of their necks, braving mud and thorns, and each other, to drop a paper sack of raspberries into my lap. From where I sat in my hospital bed, it may as well have been the moon.

I tipped the berries into my hand. Carefully. They were so soft. I studied their plump drupelets neatly stacked, their hollows pursed like lips into supple Os. Against the faded pastel of my hospital gown, the plastic, the metal, the white all around, they stood out, blood red. I ate them quickly, one by one, and let their juices dry on my hands.

I was feeling much better by then. Strange, seeing as how it had been only two weeks since the rupture. It was as though someone had pried the pain off me and simply discarded it. It was no longer mine, just a hunk of scrap metal somewhere on the bottom of the sea. My body poured back into the spaces where that pain had been. I felt full and new. Cozy, even, beneath my hospital gown and IV tubes.

There was this business of the approaching brain surgery, but in my newfound condition of painlessness, the idea was bearable. The surgery felt now like a mere formality to lock in the health that my body had already recovered. I was in no less danger. Despite my feeling so well, it was only a flimsy clot plugging the ruptured vessel that was keeping me alive. I had been told, no joke, not to sneeze.

Somehow, though, I didn't think about any of that when a nurse asked if I wanted to try standing up, maybe take a loop around the floor. I had no idea why this was even allowed, but yes, yes! I wanted to! The nurse removed my catheter and helped me to the side of the bed. The floor was perfectly flat, but when my feet touched the ground for the first time in two weeks, I felt as though I were standing on an incline. I grabbed the walker in front of me and, with a nurse on my left, Eli on my right, and someone rolling my IV behind me, I began to shuffle along.

I looked down and saw my pink traction-pad socks pulled halfway up my shins. I thought of the race in New York six weeks earlier: the opening loop around Central Park, the way we all spilled out onto Seventh Avenue and ran through an empty Times Square, the lights and billboards in full effect. I picked up speed in the final stretch down the West Side Highway. As I passed the last of the live bands, Eli and our friend Megan rode by on bikes, waving and cheering me on. It was magic.

That I'd done all that now felt like a joke. Wait, no, *this* was the joke. I laughed out loud and kept moving. My dad was there when we rounded the nurses' station. He had an odd expression on his face, as though he didn't know whether to feel relieved or heartbroken. I smiled. "I'm walking," I said, in a voice taut with childish pride. I turned away, ashamed.

After the loop came the best possible thing: a shower, an actual shower, in the nurses' changing room. My nurse wheeled me to the stall, helped me onto the shower seat, washed my hair, and then *closed the curtain*, leaving me alone with that glorious stream of hot water. It flowed onto my face and down my back. When I closed my eyes, it felt almost like real life. Back in my room, I got to sit up in a chair and comb through my hair, and put on my favorite green T-shirt instead of a gown. That's how my mom, dad, and Eli found me, clean, upright, feeling civilized, when they arrived for visiting hours with a very special package.

It was salmon, pan roasted and perfectly seasoned, from a glowy little restaurant in town called L'Amante. Eli and my dad had eaten it there the night before, and the next day they went back, determined to bring me some of my own. The chef didn't do take-out, but with the help of a sympathetic bartender, they prevailed. They'd had to "play the brain surgery card," my dad told me, and I laughed. *Brain surgery*. Even surrounded by beeping monitors and a tangle of tubes, it didn't seem possible that those words could apply to me. I dug into the plate on my lap.

The salt hit me first. For two weeks, I'd eaten nothing at all, and then only the blandest of hospital food. Lukewarm tea, flabby noodles, broccoli steamed to mush. Now, suddenly, salt! I ate and my family beamed, visibly comforted by the sight of me with this thing from the outside world. That salmon didn't belong there, and neither did I. As long as I was eating, it seemed possible that this had all been a terrible mistake.

Pan-Roasted Salmon

This is the simplest and best salmon preparation I know. I love how the skin crisps and the pink meat browns along the surface. It's the closest thing to grilled salmon, without the grill. When you purchase your fish, ask for center-cut fillets that are more or less the same thickness from end to end. And make sure to dry the salmon well before you brush the fillets with oil.

1 tablespoon flaked sea salt, like Maldon
2 pieces of salmon fillet with skin on, ⅓ pound each
Olive oil
Freshly ground black pepper and lemon wedges, for serving

Scatter the salt evenly over a dry, well-seasoned 10-inch cast-iron pan. A stainless steel pan will also work. If you're using a stainless steel pan instead of cast iron, brush the pan lightly with oil before adding the salt. Place the pan over medium-high heat for 3 minutes.

While the pan heats, dry the fish fillets well with paper towels and lay them flat on a large plate. Brush with olive oil on both sides.

Place the fish into the hot pan, skin side down. Turn the heat down slightly if the crackle sounds too loud and sputtery. Cover with a lid. If you don't have a lid that fits your pan, a metal baking sheet will do the job. Cook without moving the fillets for 3 to 5 minutes, until the skin is brown and crisp, and releases easily from the pan. Flip the fillets and cook them uncovered for another 2 to 4 minutes, depending on their thickness. The fish is done when the flesh deep inside is still faintly translucent and the internal temperature reads 125 degrees.

Serve with freshly ground black pepper and lemon wedges.

Serves 2.

CHAPTER 8

Just in Case

The summer before my junior year of college, I got a job as a resident adviser on campus so that I could afford to stay in the city (free housing!) and worked at a literary agency down in SoHo during the day. The money I made would have to stretch for course books and food that year, so to cut costs, I'd buy a head of celery and a jar of peanut butter and eat it for as many meals as I could stomach. Totally worth it for a summer on my own in New York.

On Sunday mornings, I'd strap on my Rollerblades and take off. I'd weave through street fairs, get lost in Central Park, loop around the reservoir, and pop out on the East Side. I'd stop at Fairway on my way back up to school and treat myself to a single soft-ripe peach and a couple of firmer ones for later in the week. In the evenings, I'd work on musical arrangements for the coming year. I was taking over as music director of my choir. The incoming business director was Eli.

He was in the city that summer, too, living down on Mercer Street and working as a software engineer, but for whatever reason, we didn't hang out, not once. Until one night in late August, when he met me outside my dorm to discuss choir stuff. He was sitting on the stone banister of the entryway, reading a section of the paper as I approached, and hopped down to give me a quick hug. Then he swung himself back up there, skinny legs dangling, folded the paper under his arm, and we talked.

We were pumped. He had big plans: a new website, more gigs than ever, an international tour, an album. As for me, I wanted to really push that year, get us sounding better than ever. I told him about the new music arrangements I was working on, and what I had in mind for auditions. This thing mattered to us a lot. We wanted to kill it. We were total psycho choir dorks—and we thought that was awesome. It was an amazing feeling, our mutual intensity, our desire to make something great. I climbed the stairs to my room later that night, surprisingly giddy. All I could think was, *This is going to be so good.*

It was. Eli had said right off the bat that it was his job to think of everything that needed thinking of so that I could focus on the music. He responded to e-mails, booked performance spaces, organized travel to and from gigs, and arranged for hotel rooms and home stays. We did a lot of weekends away, performing and doing music workshops with school kids, and I admired the warm, professional way he communicated with our hosts. He was so competent. So smart. I loved how much he cared. He did things exactly as I would have hoped to do them had I been running the entire show myself. No, scratch that. He did them better. Whatever I said— whatever I didn't say—Eli knew exactly what I meant, and vice versa. Someone in the group once told us that we operated like two sides of a single brain. It was true.

For two years we led the group, working hard to make music and put it out into the world, signing e-mails to each other, "your partner in crime." We'd sit next to each other on the bus rides to gigs, reviewing itineraries and set lists, then again on the way home, talking late into the night while the others dozed. "You know," his girlfriend Rebecca once said to me, "he thinks you're amazing. Beautiful, smart, fun. I mean, it's totally platonic. You never need to worry about things getting weird." I know what you're thinking. *She was his girlfriend. Of course she'd say that.* But Rebecca, she's kind of an oracle. Rebecca knows. I thought Eli was nuts when he broke things off with her.

By April of senior year, Eli had been single for a while. Things with my relationship were, well, what they'd always been. Justin felt certain that I was "it." I felt certain only that he was terrific, and after three and a half years together, it was beginning to dawn on me that terrific was maybe not enough. He was shipping off to medical school in the fall, and I was moving to England for graduate school, so I said those famous last words: "Let's take a break." And, you know, stay in touch. Visit each other on our respective continents, date some other people, see where things stand in a year.

He asked if we could carry on for the remaining few weeks of school as though we were entirely together, do all that fun senior stuff as the couple we'd always been, and I didn't see any harm, so no one knew. Except for my roommate Rachel, who also happened to sing in our choir. I'd had to tell someone.

When I explained about the sort-of split, she got quiet. She didn't mean to complicate things, she said, but had I ever thought about Eli? Was there maybe something there? I laughed until I realized she was serious. "I think he's in love with you," she said. Eli had just accepted a job in Seattle, and that's a very long way from England, Rachel pointed out. She felt she had to say something. Just in case.

Just in case what? No, I hadn't thought of it; no, there was nothing there; and no, *please no*, he couldn't be in love with me. Things would get complicated, and strained, and eventually, telling ourselves it was for the best, we'd lose touch. This was not okay. If Eli felt as Rachel suspected, we'd have to talk about it. That, or our friendship would self-destruct. I just had to get him to say it out loud. Then we could fix it.

It was a horrible plan. Not to mention cruel. Lure a friend into confessing his love for you, a friend who seems to be doing just fine keeping quiet about it, with the express purpose of rejecting him on the spot? And then what? Somehow convince him that whatever he thinks he feels, he doesn't? Yep, horrible. But never mind. Rachel was wrong. I'd confirm with Eli what I already knew—we were buds!—and we'd have a good laugh. That was what was going to happen.

I asked Eli to meet me for dinner that night at Café Pertutti on Broadway. He'd been working on a new photo project and sketched out the idea for me on a napkin while we waited for our pasta. He sucked down his water, chomped on the ice. And then slowly, casually, I started in on my search and destroy. I waited for moments when I could steer the conversation toward talk of our friendship. I tossed out line after line, setting him up to make a move. He didn't bite.

Finally, after we'd asked for the check, I told him about the thing Rebecca had said way back when, how he and I would never be more than friends. He closed his eyes for a moment, and I thought his expression half crumpled, but no, I must have imagined it, because then he looked at me straight-on and said, "Yes. That's right."

Okay, then. It was settled. We were just good friends, exactly as I suspected. Nothing would change. Perfect. A win.

Then why wasn't I relieved?

I loved him. I'd never once considered it, but there it was. I felt insane. I felt sure. I felt devastated that he didn't feel it, too, but only for a moment, because I was suddenly quite certain that he did. We paid the bill. I mumbled something about needing to pick up some sheet music from his room, and we started walking.

"Who do you think is braver?" I asked, as we approached his apartment. His cheeks flushed, and I knew he understood what I'd been asking all night long. After a pause, he said, "Maybe. With different timing, if there were no Justin, *maybe* there might have been something between us."

"And what if I told you that Justin and I are no longer together?" I spoke carefully. We were sitting on his front stoop by now. He took off his glasses and folded them in his hand. I watched him close his eyes, squeeze the bridge of his nose, and flush redder still. It was a minute or two before he spoke.

"Then I'd say I want to do my life with you," he said.

And there it was, the relief I'd been hoping for, just in a different package from the one I'd expected.

I swallowed. "Me, too."

Everything I've just said about that night, I don't believe any of it. I don't believe in feelings that sweep you away in a flash, or love without doubt, or destiny. We humans have agency. We think, and we decide, and we act. Yet that night—and I know this sounds crazy—it felt as though we had nothing to do with it. Our conversation on the steps, my words, his, they seemed to happen *to* us. It was as though we'd been setting up invisible dominoes for years without realizing it. The slightest tap, and here we were.

We stumbled around campus wide-eyed, smiling. He walked me home. The next morning, I found an e-mail from him with a single line:

"1, 2, 3, GO . . ."

And we went.

Kale and Pomegranate Salad

My mom still pokes fun at me for a phone call she received one night that week, after Eli and I made a salad together for dinner. "Mom," I said, "he cut the mushrooms just right." I had found a guy who shared my salad aesthetic, and while I admit that salad compatibility does not necessarily correlate with romantic compatibility, there is something to be said for standing at the counter together, rinsing, drying, slicing, talking about whatever, and ending up with a big bowl of salad that suits you both to a T.

Here's a salad we make as often as we can each fall while pomegranates are in season. The dressing gets its zing from pomegranate molasses, something I first tried at a Seattle restaurant called Sitka and Spruce, where they drizzle the sweet-tart syrup over yogurt and sautéed dates. The dish was genius, and I was hooked. I bought a bottle of pomegranate molasses when I got home—you can find it at Middle Eastern markets and a lot of mainstream grocery stores—and I've kept some on hand ever since. I brush it with oil over carrots and beets before roasting, add it by the tablespoon to glasses of sparkling water, spoon it over hot oatmeal, swirl it into yogurt, and whisk it into dressings like the one here.

I like my dressing on the sharp side, especially in a salad with such strong, sturdy ingredients. If you want to tone it down, add more olive oil by the teaspoon, whisking and tasting between each addition, until the balance is right for you.

One more quick note: This salad calls for dinosaur kale, the flat, dark green kind also known as lacinato or Tuscan kale. I prefer it in its raw form over curly kale, which can be tougher and harder to chew.

For the salad:

12 leaves dinosaur kale, stripped of their stems and thinly
   sliced
½ head of radicchio, thinly sliced
4 radishes, thinly sliced
Seeds from half a large pomegranate (about ½ cup)
A handful or two of roasted and salted pistachios, shelled

For the dressing:

5 tablespoons extra-virgin olive oil (plus more to taste; see
   headnote)
2 tablespoons red wine vinegar
1 tablespoon pomegranate molasses
½ teaspoon Dijon mustard

Put all the salad ingredients in a large bowl. Shake or whisk
together the dressing ingredients in a jar or mixing bowl. Depending on how heavily dressed you like your salad, you may end up with
more dressing than you need. Start with half, toss, taste, then add
more, as needed.

Serves 4.

CHAPTER 9

A Home Run

The morning of the surgery, I made Eli promise he would leave me. It was the most important thing I could think of to say in those strange few minutes alone before Patty wheeled me down. I mean, what the hell are you supposed to say, anyway? The real message, the only message, of course, is "I love you." That's all. But the weight of that moment contorts the words, makes them sound too much like "good-bye."

There was something more pressing I needed Eli to hear.

"After the surgery . . ." I began, the thought of what I was about to say tightening around my throat. "If I . . ."

"Jess, Jess—" Eli tried to cut me off.

"No, listen to me. If I wake up not me, you have to go."

I was terrified. Not of being dead, though I preferred very much not to be. The thought of death, of missing out on my life and my people, made me sad, not afraid. What I feared was something worse: being trapped in my body, being trapped outside of my own right mind, Eli feeling he must stand by me and ending up trapped as well.

"If I wake up not myself, you cannot stay."

"It's okay," he soothed. "Shhh . . ." But I knew he was with me on this. I knew he would be okay. I placed my forearms on his shoulders, locked my fingers behind the back of his neck, and as I pulled his face close, a strange mix of anguish and elation surged through me. "I love you." I was smiling and crying. "I mean it. I love you, El." That part was safe. Nothing could touch it.

Eli left the room the way he always does, opening the door just enough to slide out sideways. Patty put her hand on my back.

"You're going to be fine."

I was still unconscious when Dr. Tranmer told my family that all was well. He and his team had done just as they'd planned, sawing a several-inch hole in my skull above my left eye, locating the aneurysm, and sealing it off with a tiny clothespin of a clip like the one he'd handed me in my room. "A home run," he called it. There were hugs and high-fives all around.

When you're coming out of general anesthesia, no one takes what you have to say particularly seriously. Credibility is at an all-time low when you've been out cold for ten hours, during which time surgeons have been poking around in your brain. But something was wrong, and no one knew it yet but me.

I had opened my eyes, at least I thought I had, but the world to the left of my nose remained black. *I must be bandaged up*, I thought. *Gauze and tape must be blocking the light.* I reached through the blackness for my left eye and felt the tickle of my lashes against my finger. I blinked. I felt it again. There was no bandage, only darkness.

"I can't see out of my left eye." I said it as loudly and clearly as I could to no one in particular. A nurse came over, and I said it again.

I don't know if she didn't believe me or if she didn't understand me. Either way, she didn't seem terribly concerned. There were other people somewhere in the recovery room; I could hear them. I tried to sit up. "Please. Hello? My left eye. I can't see."

Patty met me back in my room. "You're okay, Jess," she said. "This happens sometimes. It can be hard to see when you're first waking up." She was as calm and kind as ever, and I wanted to trust her, but my vision in that eye wasn't blurry or dim. It was gone.

"No, Patty. Really. Something's wrong. I can't see." She believed me.

No one knows exactly what happened, whether my skull snapped in an awkward direction when Dr. Tranmer first went in or if, when he sealed me back up and replaced the piece of bone, it sank a little too snugly into position. What we do know is that my left optic nerve was somehow "compressed," a word that always reminds me of one of those handheld citrus presses. I've seen scans of my compressed optic nerve, and photographs of healthy ones in medical books, but I still have trouble picturing what a three-dimensional optic nerve looks like in actual space. The best I can figure is something like a peeled grape. In my case, a peeled grape now squashed between the nested cups of a citrus press.

Unlike other nerves in the human body, the optic nerve rarely heals. When it does, recovery is far from complete, but surgery to decompress the nerve can increase the chance that at least some vision will return. And so, after only an hour of consciousness, maybe two, I was back on the operating table. It would be impossible to know right away if the decompression surgery had had an effect. Any improvement would happen gradually, over months. At least this time I awoke without panic. Whatever could be done had been done.

My parents were standing over me.

"Levi," I said, "Levi." That wasn't right. That wasn't his name.
My father leaned in. "What, honey?"

I hesitated. "Eli." That was it.

"He was with you when you woke up. You don't remember," my dad explained. "He's in the waiting room with his parents. I'll get him."

I breathed in, acutely aware that I could, and when I exhaled, I felt a rush of gladness, as though a dam had broken. My own conscious mind surged out from wherever it had been, filled me to the brim. I could hear my thoughts again. That familiar internal voice, the one that chirps away at each of us, narrating our every move, I could hear it. It was me. I was me. There would be test upon test later on designed to uncover any cognitive or neurological deficits, tests that would confirm what I already knew right then: In all the ways that mattered, I was fine.

"You did great, babe." Eli was with me now. The anesthesia was wearing off. I could feel the mounting discomfort as the swelling set in and my body began the painful process of knitting itself back together. My father says that for the next twenty-four hours, I whispered only two words, "water" (to drink) and "ice" (for my head). I opened my eyes at one point to find him sitting beside me, on my right side, where people sat now so that I'd be able to see them without turning my head. My dad sat very still, just looking at me. "I've been thinking," he said. "I wish I'd had you sooner so I could know you for longer."

The next thing I remember is soup. Eli's aunt Leslie had sent up a cooler of chicken soup with my in-laws, and a few days postsurgery my mother appeared in the doorway of my room with a mugful, warmed in the nurses' microwave down the hall. I was allowed to eat before I could sit up, so a nurse rolled me over onto my right side and stuffed pillows all around to keep me there. The angle of the bed was set at a permanent forty-five degrees to increase drainage and decrease swelling. My mother smoothed a towel between my cheek and the slanted mattress. Then she spooned the first swallow of soup into my mouth. It tasted of salt and dill. Nothing like the sweet, familiar broth of my mother's chicken soup. Leslie's tasted wonderful, but foreign, and I preferred that in this strange, strange place.

Sometime that day, or maybe it was the next, Dr. Tranmer came by between visiting hours, when I was in my room alone. Dr. Tranmer is tall and tidy, a handsome man in his fifties with broad shoulders, twinkly eyes, and a quiet charisma. Warmer and kinder and more in touch with fully conscious humans than surgeons are supposed to be. He is also clearly the boss. "The General," Eli called him. I was glad he was in charge.

He pulled a chair up to my bed as he always did, scooted in close, propped one foot up on a nearby chair, and leaned back. This was his signature position, how he spoke with me every time. It was a comically casual stance, especially when he was dressed in scrubs. It was like seeing your famous history professor at home in his pajamas. Only instead of weird, it was reassuring.

"I'm very sorry about your eye, Jess," he said quietly.

I couldn't believe it. I could hardly bear it, actually. This man had just dragged me from a tank of sharks and here he was apologizing for scraping my knee on the way up.

"You saved me." My voice sounded all stretched out. "Thank you."

I asked him what it would be like, having only one eye. I wanted to know if I'd be able to read, to type my dissertation.

He brightened. "Oh, yes." The biggest challenge, he explained, would be impaired depth perception. You need both eyes to perceive depth at close range. I'd already noticed the impairment. When my mother had handed me a napkin to wipe the soup from my chin, I'd reached for it and missed. Beyond several feet, Dr. Tranmer went on, depth perception isn't a binocular phenomenon. Driving, then, was still as safe as ever for me. He said my brain would sort things out with time. "Even if you never regain any sight in your left eye, your vision will improve," he said. "So much so, that one day you probably won't even notice a deficit."

Sweet and Clear Chicken Soup

With all due respect and deepest gratitude for Aunt Leslie's chicken soup, the soup I make at home is my mother's. There are two defining features of her soup, both oft discussed around my childhood table: sweetness and clarity. The sweetness is thanks to the parsnip. The clarity, well, it depends whom you ask.

My mother begins by washing her chicken under cold water and plucking out visible feathers. She then plunges the chicken, a couple of pieces at a time, into a pot of boiling water to remove any remaining blood. Next, she plucks out more pinfeathers, the little ones that are now sticking up from the heat. "I don't take the time to remove *all* the feathers," she insists. That would be excessive. (Her mother, she says, removed every last one.) My mother then empties and cleans the pot and . . . starts the soup.

Honestly, my mother's soup is so good that if all these steps were the only way, the effort would be worth it. But I certainly wouldn't make it very often. Fortunately, I've found another, abbreviated route to a soup that's just as clear. (Really. My mom has given it her blessing!)

For a clear, golden soup my way, all you have to do is cook it uncovered, at a very low simmer, and skim, skim, skim. Never let it boil, which would cause the fat and blood remnants to emulsify and cloud the broth.

Growing up, we always ate this soup with fine egg noodles and matzo balls. Today I'm just as likely to spoon in some of whatever cooked grain I have left over in the fridge: rice, farro, barley. They all do the trick.

1 yellow onion, peeled

6 carrots, peeled

2 parsnips, peeled

5 celery stalks

1 3- to 4-pound chicken, cut up into pieces, giblets removed (you may buy a cut-up chicken, if you prefer)

1 tablespoon Diamond Crystal kosher salt, plus more for cooking the vegetables

A few extra carrots, parsnips, and celery stalks (3 to 4 of each to serve 8 people)

2–3 cups cooked egg noodles, rice, farro, or barley

Slice a deep X into the top of the onion, but don't cut all the way through. You want the onion to remain whole. Cut the carrots, parsnips, and celery into 1-inch pieces. Put all the vegetables into an 8-quart stock pot, add the chicken pieces, and sprinkle with the tablespoon of salt. Cover with cold water (about 4 quarts), and slowly bring to the barest possible simmer. Do not cover the pot. Do not let boil.

Start skimming the surface of the broth with a spoon as soon as there's something to skim, and keep skimming as foam, fat, and blood rise to the surface. You want to catch what comes up before it has a chance to sink back into the soup and emulsify. For 20 to 30 minutes, you'll be skimming like crazy, then just every so often until the soup is done. Cook at a low, low simmer for 2 hours total, then remove the pot from the heat.

Transfer the chicken from the pot to a plate. Line a fine-meshed sieve with cheesecloth and place it over a large bowl or container. Ladle the soup and its vegetables into the bowl through the cloth-lined sieve. You can skip the sieving if you want and simply remove the vegetables. The broth will still be beautiful and delicious. (Just don't tell my mom.) Discard the vegetables. Cover and refrigerate the broth overnight.

Once the chicken is cool enough to handle, remove the meat from the bones, shred with your fingers, and store in the fridge separate from the broth. When you're ready to serve the soup, remove the shredded chicken from the fridge and bring a medium-sized saucepan of water to a boil. Add a few pinches of salt to the water. Peel the extra carrots and parsnips, slice them and the celery into 1-inch pieces, and cook in the boiling water for 3 to 5 minutes, until they're soft enough to pierce easily with a fork, but still firm. Meanwhile, remove the broth from the fridge and skim off any fat floating on the surface. Reheat the broth in a pot. Add some shredded chicken, vegetables, and whichever rice, noodle, or grain you prefer to individual soup bowls, ladle in the broth, and serve.

Serves 8.

CHAPTER 10

The Most Beautiful Things

We didn't kiss that night on the steps of Eli's apartment. In fact, we didn't kiss anyplace for ten whole days. I felt terrible enough as it was about these feelings that had unfurled like sails. I tried to explain to Justin what had happened, as though it were something I could explain: how unexpected that conversation with Eli had been, how fishy it looked, I knew, that I'd suggested a break and now this. Justin stared at me serenely. "It's okay," he said. *It was?* "You're confused." College was over, I was moving far away, he figured. He thought I was going through a thing. Maybe he was right. But I didn't think so.

It was the end of the semester. We were squeezing in last choir concerts and extra rehearsals for the album we were recording, spending tens of hours each week in the studio. I saw Eli almost every day. We didn't tell our friends that anything had changed, and by all outward appearances, nothing had. In between concerts, rehearsals, and studio sessions, I'd convince myself I had made the whole thing up. I wasn't in love. Then Eli would walk into the room: "Hey, lady." Oh, right, I was. We were.

One Sunday, our recording session in the studio ran especially long. It was 9:00 p.m. by the time we left after twelve hours of recording. I went straight home to sleep. Eli did, too, but he decided that first he needed to eat. He put up a pot of water to boil, cooked himself some pasta, and went to drain it into a colander in the sink when, exhausted and low on blood sugar, he poured its entire contents over his forearm.

His roommate called an ambulance, and by the time my phone rang after midnight, Eli was home again, all bandaged up. There was a prescription for Tylenol with codeine waiting for him at the pharmacy that his roommate had offered to pick up.

"No, I'll get it," I said. "I'm coming over."

Eli was lying on his bed, propped up by a few pillows, when I arrived. I handed him his water bottle and unscrewed the cap on the Tylenol. I sat down on the bed. We talked for a bit; he told me about the medics and how, according to protocol, they'd asked, "Do you remember what happened?" How he nearly laughed out loud when he said, "Yes, I poured boiling hot water on my arm!" I got up to leave as he started to drift off, then turned back and hugged him. His face was red, and very close to mine. I knew what was coming. I hoped I knew.

"I want to give you a kiss," he said, "but I'm not sure you want me to."

"I want you to."

And he did. On the *forehead*. That probably sounds terribly anticlimactic and chaste, but I'm telling you, it was perfect. I felt as though my limbs were about to fly off my body. I had no idea a kiss could even feel that way. A kiss on the forehead, no less.

Eli ran into Rebecca the following week at a party.

"I'm seeing someone new," he told her.

"Jessica," she said.

"How did you know?"

She smiled. "It's perfect."

Eli's mother, Sarah, would no doubt like me to mention here that she knew it all along. She'd prayed for it.

When Eli and I first started directing our choir, we held a group retreat at the Schleifers' house. They made us feel right at home, filling our bellies with chicken soup and roast beef the night we arrived and letting us rehearse for hours in their living room. Sarah likes to remind me that she had a feeling about the girl in the long gray skirt, the one waving her hands and stopping the group mid-song to give notes. She never said a word to Eli for years, but when he told her we were together, she screamed and clapped her hands and leaped into the air.

After graduation, before his move to Seattle in early July, Eli lived with his parents. I needed a place near the city to stay as we finished up the album, so I joined him. He slept in "the boys' room" with one of his brothers who was also home that summer, and I bunked with his sister across the hall. Every morning for two weeks, we'd wake up early and meet down at the table for a quick breakfast of cold cereal and orange juice. Eli's father, Steve, had procured an enormous, four-pound box of Grape-Nuts, my favorite. Eli ate Life cereal, and quickly. Once you've poured the milk, he explained, you don't have long before it sogs. It was here where I learned that there would be no breakfast conversation on Life cereal days. "I've poured the milk," Eli says, to this day, if I utter anything that requires a reply.

After breakfast, Eli's father would drop us at the Route 4 shuttle stop on his way to work. We'd ride across the bridge to the George Washington terminal, Eli's hand resting on my thigh while he read the *New York Times*, and take the train to the studio from there.

On Saturday afternoon I got my first taste of Sarah's weekly cholent. Cholent—pronounced with a *ch* like "cherry"—is a long-simmered stew of meat, barley, potatoes, and beans that's traditionally served for lunch on the Jewish Sabbath, when cooking is prohibited. Cholent works around the restriction by getting its start in the pot on Friday afternoon, before the Sabbath begins, then cooking slowly on its own over low heat all through the night. That way, observant Jews can still eat a hot meal for Sabbath lunch, a religious obligation according to some, and in any case nice to have. The word "cholent" derives from the Latin *calentem*, meaning "that which is hot." But there's a folk etymology I love: Why is it called "cholent"? Because of its French pronunciation, which sounds like the French words for "warm" and "slow": *chaud, lent.*

Cholent has been around for centuries, and there are variations all over the world. Some go by different names: the Middle Eastern *hamin* made with chicken and rice, the Moroccan *s'hina* with chickpeas and hulled wheat, turmeric, and cumin. Sometimes eggs are buried beneath the stew and left to cook in their shells.

The lineage of Sarah's cholent is eastern European, where meat, potatoes, beans, and barley were the norm, flavored with onion, salt, and pepper. In the Polish town where Sarah's mother grew up, homes had only small, wood-burning ovens that would grow cold over the Sabbath, when it was forbidden to stoke the fire. So on Friday before sundown, someone from each family would carry the cholent pot to the baker's large oven, which, even untended, retained enough heat to cook the entire town's worth of cholents overnight. Once all the pots were inside, the oven would be sealed until after the Sabbath service the following day, when people would pick up their cholents and carry them home for lunch.

Sarah prepares hers as her mother did, with a thick batter of flour, eggs, and onion poured on top of the cholent once it's hot. It steams and cooks through under the lid of the pot to form a savory cake, a "cholent kugel," that tastes of the beans and meat stewing beneath it. It's Eli's favorite part.

When the cholent came around at that first lunch, Eli urged me to grab some kugel. I said okay, but I must not have been moving quickly enough, because he suddenly dug into the pot, fished out a hunk, and plopped it down on my plate with such energy that it splattered sauce onto the tablecloth. "There," he said, satisfied, as though he'd just kept the kugel from making its great escape.

My twenty-second birthday fell the next day, on the Sunday of Memorial Day weekend. Eli wanted to help his parents clean out their basement and build wall-to-wall shelving for the remaining stuff before he moved. Looking back, this is not an activity that's exactly celebratory, but I couldn't imagine a better way to spend the day.

We sorted old photos into boxes. Sarah on her wedding day, with straight hair halfway down her back and a center part; an Alaskan malamute named Mookie; a miniature Eli, serious and unsmiling in every shot. There were large canvases filled with his brother's paintings, Eli's childhood mug collection, and a graveyard of suitcases with jammed zippers, broken wheels, and missing straps. I loved every second. I loved digging through the history of the family that I was shyly beginning to think of as mine.

Once we'd cleared enough space along the back wall, we started building the shelves. I'm terrible with a hammer, so Eli had me work the ratchet. I liked the sound it made as the pawl clicked through the gear. Eli noticed and smiled. "Ratch, ratch, ratch," he whispered. I felt my chest and cheeks go hot.

A month to the day earlier, I'd come up out of the Lincoln Center subway stop to find a building completely demolished. The brick face of the building beside it was now exposed, painted top to bottom with an advertisement for Hunter Baltimore Rye. It was faded in places, but the adjacent building had shielded it from too much damage. The colors were bright, blue and red letters against a taxicab yellow. A man in a red riding coat sat atop a horse, midstrut. He had a handlebar mustache and was tipping his hat. I joined a few others on the sidewalk, staring, before ducking into the lobby of the building next door and asking the older gentleman at the desk about it.

He had all kinds of stories. The building had once been Liberty Warehouse Storage, he said, which had specialized in pianos, furniture, and art. There had been hydraulic elevators inside large enough to fit these things and the horses that transported them. The horses would deliver their goods, then continue on up to the top floor to board.

I e-mailed Eli right away. This long-buried layer of New York, unearthed by the remaking and rebuilding of the city around it: Wasn't it amazing? A building collapsed, and there it was.

Without telling me, Eli had gone down to photograph the site with his brother's Yashica-Mat. My birthday gift that year was a framed fourteen-by-fourteen-inch print of the painted building against a clear blue sky. He inscribed the back in red Sharpie:

"The most beautiful things are all around us. You just need to look."

Sarah's Cholent with Kugel

The nuts and bolts of this cholent are Sarah's mother's. When Sarah got married and moved to suburban New Jersey, she made some changes, following the lead of her neighbors. "We added the American stuff,"

Sarah explained when I asked her for the recipe. "The tomato sauce." (I nodded.) "The beef bouillon." (I wrote it down.) "The onion soup mix." *The what?* It's true. This cholent is a mere whisper of itself without a packet of Goodman's onion soup mix (I've tried), so don't skip it.

Like Sarah, I make this cholent in a 6-quart slow cooker. While everything in the pot will be cooked through and very likely delicious after 5 to 10 hours, you need the full 18 to 24 hours for the flavors and texture to come together as intended.

For the cholent:

  1 large yellow onion, coarsely chopped

  2 tablespoons olive oil

  3 pounds flanken (bone-in short ribs) or stew meat

  1 packet Goodman's onion soup mix

  2 potatoes (I use 1 baking potato and 1 sweet potato)

  ⅓ cup each dried pinto beans, red kidney beans, and navy
      beans

  ½ cup barley

  1 15-ounce can tomato sauce, preferably Muir Glen

  1 beef bouillon cube, preferably Telma, dissolved in 2 cups
      hot water

For the kugel:

  5 large eggs

  2 tablespoons canola oil

  ¼ cup water

  1 large onion

  2¼ cups (281 grams) all-purpose flour

  A generous pinch of fine sea salt

  Freshly ground black pepper

Assemble the cholent:

Put the chopped onion into a 6-quart slow cooker and cover with the olive oil. Turn the pot on to its lowest, slowest setting. (It's the ten-hour setting on mine.) Lay the meat on top of the onion, and cover evenly with the onion soup mix. Peel the potatoes, cut each one into eighths, and arrange them on top of the meat in a ring against the sides of the pot. Fill the center of the potato ring with the beans and the barley, and dump the can of tomato sauce on top. Pour in the water with the dissolved bouillon cube, then add water until the ingredients are just barely covered. Be sure to leave enough room at the top of the pot for the kugel. Do not stir. Cover the pot.

Make the kugel:

Two to three hours into cooking, once the cholent is quite hot, whisk together the eggs, oil, and water in a large bowl. Coarsely grate in as much of the onion as you can without hurting your fingers, add the salt, a few grinds of black pepper, and stir. Add the flour, a little at a time, and stir until a loose dough forms and pulls away from the sides of the bowl. Pour the kugel dough into the center of the cholent. It will spread some as it cooks. If you notice that your water level is low, add some more. Cover, and cook for 18 to 24 hours.

To serve, lift the kugel out of the pot and slice it into squares. Spoon the cholent with its juices into a large casserole dish, then pile the kugel squares on top.

Serves 8 or more.

CHAPTER 11

Riptide

I closed the eye that worked and strained into the resulting darkness. I tried to look around inside of it for something, anything, but there was only black. When the panic hit, my right eye flew open and the room sprang back into perfect position, like a page from a pop-up book. I caught my breath, then closed my seeing eye again and thrust myself back into darkness. And again and again. I couldn't help myself. I was checking, I guess. Can I see something now? *Now?*

It was Sunday, three days after the surgeries, and I was sitting up in bed. My E.T. finger, the one that glowed red from the taped-on oxygen sensor, was on my left hand. I reached across my face with it to the side of the world that showed up. Then I pulled my hand leftward and stared straight ahead as my glowing fingertip disappeared over the bridge of my nose like a tiny sunset. I was playing with my new body the way you play with a new toy, figuring out which button does something cool and which one does nothing at all.

According to my father, I'd returned to a room in the ICU one over from the one I'd left. I hadn't believed him. There were the chocolates and seltzer bottles lined up on the windowsill in the same order they had been. There was that creepy stuffed flower, propped up against the wall by the sink. My black sketch pad was just where I kept it on the bedside table, and beside it was my pen.

"Patty arranged the new room for you so that it would look exactly the same," my father explained.

I was furious. It was the kindest gesture, but it felt like a trick. I wasn't angry at Patty. I was angry at myself for falling for it. That I couldn't tell the difference terrified me. Was it the missing field of vision that threw me? Or had my brain been damaged in surgery after all? I was mad at my body and tired.

Eli called late that afternoon from New York. He'd just finished his hundred-mile ride and he was tired, too, but good tired. Great tired. He sounded like himself for the first time in weeks. I felt as though someone had slid open a manhole cover at last and lowered the phone down to where I lay stuck underground. I pressed the receiver to my ear with both hands.

Eli told me about the rain thumping against the car's windshield and the speeding ticket he had earned as he'd hightailed it away from Burlington. I pictured him making his getaway, driving as fast as he could with his bike strapped to the trunk. He told me about the crush at the starting line, how the space between riders gradually equalized and each rider pedaled on, as if in his own invisible chute. Eli began the ride with our friend Megan, but they split up early on. Some miles in, he and another man fell into pace. One would pull ahead and the other would fall back, then they'd wordlessly switch. They rode at least fifty miles that way. All the way through, Eli's legs never protested. At the end he was happy, and ready for a cold beer. I wanted to clap a bell jar down over him there, let him stay in that space for a while as I looked on.

Earlier that summer, just before we'd left for New York, I'd gotten my first road bike. It was a birthday gift from Eli, who was excited for me to join him on his rides. I'd never ridden a bike with drop handle-bars or the kind of pedals you have to clip into with special shoes. We'd practiced that summer in a park on the Lower East Side. More than once, I'd rolled to a stop, tried and failed to free my foot from the pedal, and tipped over onto the ground, still one with the bike. I would stand up, laughing, and get back on. From my hospital bed I wondered if I'd ever feel safe on a bike again, now that half of my world had gone black.

One of my last days in the ICU, Dr. Tranmer stopped by to explain what would happen next. Eli was back from New York now. He stood by my bed, while Dr. Tranmer assumed his usual position, slouched in one chair with his leg propped up on another. He folded a sheet of paper to stiffen it for writing, laid it against his thigh, and drew us the blood vessel and its attendant aneurysm as he'd done before the surgery. Again, he penned the straight wall of the vessel, then the aneurysm ballooning outward from it in the shape of a kidney bean. Only now, he added another line across the base of the aneurysm, separating it from the vessel. This was the clip. He ran the pen back and forth a couple of times so that the clip stood out in bold. Until he pointed it out, we didn't notice that he hadn't drawn it flush against the vessel. There was a sliver of the aneurysm still beneath it.

A residual aneurysm is common after clipping a bean-shaped aneurysm, he explained. Most likely, the clip would stay firmly in place and the minor deformity of the vessel would spend the rest of its days unchanged until I died an old woman. (Peacefully, in my sleep, arm in arm with Eli, of course.)

There was unfortunately also the chance that pressure would build beneath the clip and a new aneurysm would form out of the bit that remained. It would need to be monitored. That meant an angiogram every six months for a year, then yearly for five years, then every five years after that.

Okay. But how was I supposed to understand all of this in terms of my actual life? That was what I wanted to know. Was it safe to run? How far? How fast? Was pregnancy an option for me? When? These questions were impossible to answer, but Dr. Tranmer spoke kindly and did his best. Pregnancy would probably be safe one day, though it was too soon to say so for sure. Pushing would not. I looked at Eli and tried to read his face. It had taken us years to know with certainty that we wanted to be parents. The feeling of sureness was still new. Maybe I could make myself not want it anymore. I groped around for the old familiar doubt, but I couldn't find it.

"No marathons," Dr. Tranmer went on. "The occasional short run should be fine." But how occasional was occasional? How short was short? Three miles? Five? What do words like "probably" and "should be" even mean when the potential reality that lies beyond them is death?

Dr. Tranmer was in one-step-at-a-time mode, the only mode appropriate after brain surgery, when the body is just beginning to heal and the first follow-up scan is still six months away. I, on the other hand, wanted an operating manual, and a lifetime warranty to boot. What *exactly* do I need to do to make sure I'll be okay?

My official prognosis, it seemed, was that I was going to be either absolutely fine or not, based either entirely or not at all on whether I crossed certain red lines, sketchily drawn—that may or may not be red lines at all. This is the prognosis of every human, of course, from the healthy and strong to the gravely ill, every single moment of our lives. We forget that. (And thank goodness.) One inconvenience of having just been nearly dead was that I could no longer help but remember.

I moved out of the ICU and onto a regular floor that night. Eli was sitting at the foot of my bed when an e-mail came in on his phone.

"Josh and Melissa are splitting up." He said it before he'd had a chance to process the news himself, and from his offhand tone I was sure I'd misheard.

"What?"

These friends of ours had been together for ten years, married for six. We'd met them for drinks before leaving New York a few weeks earlier. They had just bought a place in the city. In another year, they told us, they were hoping to have a child.

"No," I sobbed. "No, no, no . . ." Everything was broken. This was too much. I kicked at the sheets and pounded the mattress with my fists.

"You have to calm down," my father said gently, but I couldn't. For the first time since I'd fallen from the treadmill, I cried with all my might. Eli was with me on the bed now. I flung myself at him, tucked myself into a ball on his lap with my knees up under my chin and my face pressed into his chest. Then, out of nowhere, a riptide of gratitude.

"I am the luckiest," I croaked into Eli's T-shirt between ragged breaths. "I have everything. I am the luckiest one."

Before Eli left for the night he leaned in close to my head, a changed landscape with its ear-to-ear stitches along a strip of bald scalp, its temples swollen and bruised. I knew the forehead kiss was coming, but the nerves had been cut. I couldn't feel his lips at all.

CHAPTER 12

Plotting, Together

"**M**ake sure you get a window seat on the left side of the plane," Eli told me. He'd been living in Seattle for two months, and I was flying out to visit him for the first time. He wanted me to see Mt. Rainier as the plane passed by. I was afraid I would miss it, so once we crossed the Mississippi, I barely peeled my eyes from the window. You get far enough west, and lots of mountaintops pop up through the clouds. I wasn't sure I'd know which one was Rainier. Eli assured me that I would.

Truly, there was no mistaking it. The peak was enormous, grand, snow swept, catching the light along its slopes and grooves. The contours of the rock appeared sketched and shaded in with pencil. In fact, the whole mountain seemed drawn, painted, the backdrop for a movie set. Framed by my tiny bubble of a window it looked like something I could hold in my hand.

Eli picked me up from the airport and we drove to the little apartment he'd found in Capitol Hill. It was our first time really alone, ever. This visit would be our last before I moved to England for graduate school, and we were determined to make the most of it. We wandered from Eli's place down to Pike Place Market and ate Beecher's grilled cheese sandwiches by Puget Sound. We climbed to the top of the water tower in Volunteer Park, then snacked on chocolate-covered cherries in the grass. My dad had given me an old fully manual film camera for college graduation, and I shot my first rolls on that trip. While Eli was at work, I wandered the neighborhood, grateful for the weight of the camera around my neck and the click, whirr, click that told me I was indeed right there.

At the end of my stay, we hiked up along the White Chuck River and spent a few days camping near Glacier Peak. I awoke in our tent on the first morning to find Eli peering out at me over the top of his sleeping bag.

"I'm thinking about the ring I want to make for you," he said. "It's beautiful."

I didn't know what to say, or what to do with myself, so I pulled the sleeping bag closed over my face, curled up like a potato bug, and butted him in the shoulder with my head. Then I poked my face out, and we lay there for a while in silence, listening to the rain on the leaves.

I was so glad for that visit. This way, I could picture Eli in his space, doing his thing, as I scratched off phone cards from half a world away. When I thought of Eli, I thought of Seattle, and vice versa. I'd travel back there a few times over the next two years, first from England, and then from Israel, where I lived during my second year abroad. And when I finally bought a one-way ticket back to the U.S.A., it was to Seattle. The city already felt like home.

I've often felt as though Seattle were in on some kind of secret back then, a secret about who we were, who we would become, and the life that would be ours. Seattle is the city where Eli learned how to climb mountains (he'd summit Mt. Rainier years later), how to build big things out of wood, and where I ran my first 5K. It's where we started plotting, together, the rest of our lives.

It's also where I lived, for the first time, in an apartment all my own and learned that from inside of me, and me alone, I could spin this thing called home. My place was just a couple of blocks from Eli's and I saw him most days, but I loved living alone. Just me and my green-and-yellow-tiled kitchen, my bedroom window that I could climb out of onto a wooden balcony, and my copious closet space, most of which remained empty, since at twenty-four, I didn't yet have much stuff. I bought a kitchen table for twenty-five dollars from a woman whose husband had made it in college. I wrote the lesson plans there for the fifth grade class I was teaching and served my first solo-hosted meal there: cream of asparagus soup, zucchini quiche, and a baguette that I picked up from a bakery in Pike Place Market and stuffed with butter, garlic, and thyme. I didn't have a blender, so I borrowed Eli's to purée the soup, a soup I liked so much that I bought myself an immersion blender for all the puréeing I knew was yet to come. It was the first kitchen tool with a motor I'd ever owned. (Also, at twenty bucks, the first I could afford.)

One morning in April, three Aprils after that first conversation on his dormitory steps, and nine months after I moved to Seattle, Eli told me to meet him by his car. He wouldn't say where we were going. I should have known that something special was about to happen—he isn't usually one for surprises—but I didn't have a clue.

We parked on First Avenue, about a block from Pike Place Market, and Eli led me into a storefront I'd never noticed before. There was jewelry on display, and suddenly I understood. He'd picked out a ring. He was about to propose. I'd forgotten about our conversation in the tent by the river, the ring he said he'd mapped out in his mind. I still didn't remember when he introduced me to John, who looked more like a craftsman than a salesman, nor did I remember when John guided us behind the counter and handed Eli a small metal box. Eli opened it and removed a ring made of green wax, and that was when I got it. He hadn't *picked out* a ring. This was the model for the ring he had *designed*.

"So . . ." he said, "what do you say?"

We cast the ring together.

We wanted a fall wedding, and six months later, on October 30, we had one. We were moving to Cambridge, Massachusetts, where I'd been accepted into graduate school, so we decided to have the wedding not far from there, right outside of Boston, on the North Shore. My family came from Ohio, and his from New Jersey, and close friends from all over.

The first snow of the season fell the night before the wedding, but by morning the temp had reached the midseventies, so we moved the ceremony outdoors and set up the chuppah facing the ocean. There was French toast and bluegrass and baskets filled with pomegranates, and several ladybugs that found their way into my veil. I could say more about that day, but I want to rewind a bit, to a morning in July a few months earlier, July 14, to be exact, when Eli and I went down to the Seattle courthouse and got married, just us.

I refer to it now as "our first wedding," though when we set out for the courthouse that day, we didn't see it as a real marriage at all. I just needed a few months of health insurance between the end of my teaching job and the start of graduate school. I'd be going on Eli's plan once we were married, anyway, so why not? Let's get civilly married here in Seattle, right now, we figured, and save the thousands of dollars in Cobra fees. It was a formality, that was all. The real wedding would be the ceremony a few months later, with a rabbi and a long white dress and all the people we loved best.

It was a Thursday morning, and we went down to the courthouse first thing. I wore a cream linen skirt and a green shirt with a small pineapple embroidered on the breast. Eli wore jeans and a black tee. We waited in line for the license and got our time slot with the judge. We were visibly nonchalant and giggly, and when we told the clerk that we were there without witnesses or rings, she looked at us hard, as though we should maybe take some time to think through this decision and come back when we were responsible adults. We told her that we didn't mind paying the fee to hire two witnesses on the spot, then dashed downstairs to the kiosk in the lobby to find something in place of rings to exchange. We chose a FireBall, for Eli, and a Lemonhead, for me.

A few minutes later, Judge Richard D. Eadie married us, with a clerk and a secretary, our paid witnesses, standing solemnly by. We explained more than once that, honestly, we didn't care which ceremony from the giant binder Judge Eadie read. He could pick it himself. Really. Just choose the shortest one. Eli had to get to work.

We stood on either side of Judge Eadie clutching our penny candy. I spoke first, reading the words from the laminated binder sheet. Even the shortest, simplest script included some basic things about love, a lifetime of it, commitment, and a version of 'til death do us part. That was fine. No big deal. We were only stating the obvious. But in the presence of a judge and two witnesses, standing face-to-face and saying these words out loud felt unexpectedly powerful. Eli gave me the hairy eyeball when my voice started to shake—this wasn't our actual wedding!—but his face softened as he, too, began to hear the words, feel them, and know that they were real. When it was his turn, his voice shook, too.

We left the courthouse hand in hand, me sucking the Lemonhead, he the FireBall. We kissed with candy breath and he drove off to work. I stuffed the candy wrapper into my skirt pocket. Then I made my way to Pike Place Market to replenish my cheese supply. It was early for lunch, but I was suddenly ravenous. I bought a grilled cheese sandwich from the shop and found a spot on the grassy hill overlooking Puget Sound. The fog was burning off by now and the eastern slopes of the Olympic Mountains came into view. Ferries set out for the islands, a ship steered into the harbor, and orange cranes stretched their dinosaur necks toward the sky.

Cream of Asparagus Soup

I like crème fraîche as the "cream" in this soup for its extra tang, but heavy cream here is also lovely. The soup improves after a night in the fridge, so I recommend making it in advance. Reheat it before adding the lemon juice.

> 1 large yellow onion
> 2 pounds asparagus stalks, their tough bottoms snapped off
> 2 tablespoons unsalted butter
> Diamond Crystal kosher salt and freshly ground black pepper
> 4–5 cups vegetable broth
> ½ cup crème fraîche or heavy cream
> 1 teaspoon fresh-squeezed lemon juice

Coarsely chop the onion. Cut the asparagus into 1- to 2-inch pieces.

Melt the butter in a 4-quart pot over medium-low heat, add the onion, and cook, stirring, until softened. Add the asparagus pieces, a couple of pinches of salt and a few grinds of black pepper, and cook, stirring occasionally, for 5 minutes. Add 4 cups of vegetable broth and simmer, partially covered, until the asparagus is very ten-der, 15 to 20 minutes.

Purée the soup in batches in a stand blender, or use an immer-sion blender to purée it in the pot. (If you go the stand blender route, wait for the soup to cool a bit and fill the blender only one-half to three-quarters of the way full with each batch. Return the puréed soup to the pot.) Stir in the crème fraîche or heavy cream, then add up to another cup of broth, if necessary, to thin the soup to the consistency you prefer. If you refrigerate the soup overnight, you'll likely want to add the additional broth before reheating.

Taste, and season with salt and pepper. Stir in the lemon juice just before serving.

Serves 4.

CHAPTER 13

The Everywhere Light

Agrocery list is a crystal ball of sorts. You sit down with an empty page and see your table, your lunchbox, your pie plate as they soon will be. A list is pure potential. It means believing in the future, that there is one, and you're in it. It means getting to think about what sounds good, beyond what you're hungry for now to what you might like tomorrow.

I spent my last days at Fletcher Allen hospital making lists. "Food, first week home," I wrote at the top of a blank white page. I wasn't hungry, but that was beside the point. Sooner or later I would be, and I wanted to be ready.

I organize my grocery lists by department: produce, dairy, center aisles, specialty. My stepmom, Amy, taught me this trick for moving through the store at maximum speed, crossing off items in order. Part list, part map, it's wonderfully efficient. In the hospital, I watched the words appear in my handwriting, the letters slanting and curling in their familiar way, and had the sense that I was tracing, guiding my pen along the grooves of the lists I'd made so many times before. Only this was no ordinary list. I was plotting my escape.

carrots
kale
green apples

yogurt, 2%
milk
sharp cheddar

sardines
rice cakes
almond butter

olives (with pits)

In the bottom right corner of the page I listed my favorite breakfasts and drew a box around them.

crispy rice and eggs
oatmeal
toast with tahini and honey

I'd coax myself back to the table with these things. Surrounded by what she liked to eat before, that same person was bound to turn up.

Here on a normal floor of the hospital, for normal patients, dressed in my own pajamas instead of a johnny, I figured the rest of my recovery would look familiar. Like those draggy days after a stomach bug, maybe, or the end of a bad cold. I was surprised when Dr. Tranmer suggested rehab.

"Just for a week or so," he said. "To get your strength back. You'll love it there. It's like a hotel."

The day the two nurses arrived to transport me to the rehab center was not a good one. Or maybe it was just a bad hour. It was like that, one moment sitting up in bed, giddy with thoughts of the produce aisle, the next, nauseated, curled on one side, so heavy with exhaustion I thought the bed might give way.

The nurses strapped me to a wheelchair like a piece of cargo. They lifted my hands and legs into place and draped a blanket over my knees. I let them. I was a lump. Dead weight. My arms were free, but they felt tied into their position, one folded on top of the other across my lap. One of the nurses came around behind me, grabbed the handles of the wheelchair, and we were off, fast. Past patient rooms with open doors, past nurses' stations and orderlies stacking meal trays into carts. There was an elevator, double doors, and then, for the first time in a month, I was outside.

I lowered my eyelids to half-mast and tilted my chin toward my chest. Daylight was different from indoor light. There was more of it, and it came from everywhere. It *was* everywhere. Except for where it wasn't, the conspicuous black hole where the world on my left was supposed to be. I hated that darkness more in the everywhere light of day.

The nurse rolled me into a van that smelled of cigarette smoke. I thought of my grandmother Louise. This was the way she'd traveled after her stroke, in a van with a wheelchair slot. The nurses locked my chair down into the floor the way I'd watched my grandfather do so many times. I felt as though my body had calcified into a hard shell, so rigid that I could climb right out and leave an intact fossil behind. When the van turned, the chair tugged against its anchors, and I feared it would come loose and tip me onto the floor. A few minutes later, we were there. The nurse wheeled me inside. It smelled like a nursing home, medicinal, sterile, musty with the odor of sick people. It smelled like freezer burn.

As far as rehab centers go, it wasn't bad. It was clean. The people were nice. Still. I wouldn't need my shopping list there.

We passed some patients as the nurse wheeled me to my room in the brain injury wing. A guy in his early twenties was wearing a metal brace like a cage around his torso. It connected to a pole that ran along the back of his neck, which in turn connected to several bowed pieces flush against his scalp. Rods shot out of the contraption from there, up and over his head, like a crown. He jerked down the hallway with his legs in a too-wide stance and his arms out to the sides. Someone else walked with a bar across his shoulders that seemed intended to help him balance. Another person was in a wheelchair with her face drooping off to one side. A couple of patients had guards sitting outside their doors to make sure they didn't leave.

These were my neighbors in the neuro wing. I did not want to be these people. I did not want even to be in the same category as these people. And I wasn't, not really. But I'd come awfully close.

I soon realized that I was in the best shape of anyone there. Not because of anything I had or hadn't done. What happened, what hadn't, what could have, what should have—none of it had been up to me. The thought terrified more than it comforted: My health was as much a fluke as the next person's illness.

"Whoa," people would say when they heard my story. "You're one lucky girl." They were right, of course. But the relief in their pronouncements unnerved me. There was a ring of finality to them, as though I'd fortuitously stumbled to the side just as a runaway truck barreled past, and I could now go on my merry way. I was still so in it, though. At once wishing myself away from the mess I was in, and throbbing with gratitude that I was there to wish anything at all.

My room looked just like the hospital room I'd left not an hour before. Same stiff sheets, same blanket, same sink by the foot of the bed with the same antibacterial soap dispenser fastened to the wall. The only difference was that, now, I shared a bathroom with a diarrheal logging accident victim one room over. This was no hotel.

A nurse helped me onto the bed. I sat sidesaddle, with my feet dangling a few inches off the floor. A neurologist came in and ran me through the usual tests, shining lights in my eyes, having me touch my nose with one finger, then the other, with my eyes open and closed. "Follow me," he said, slapping his thigh with his palms a few times, then with the backs of his hands, then alternating between the two, front back, front back, faster, faster. I did what he did and for a few seconds we slapped away together, like something out of a Three Stooges routine. I felt a laugh creeping up on me, pressing itself against my pursed lips. I looked over at my parents, who had just arrived. They were smirking, too, and my laugh pushed its way out.

The day I checked into rehab was a Friday. My mom would be heading back home to Cleveland that afternoon. First, though, she would help me take a shower. I hadn't had one since the surgery, since I'd lost the vision in my left eye.

She wheeled me down the hallway to the shower room, spread a towel on the plastic seat beneath the showerhead, and helped me undress. She turned on the water and lowered me onto the seat.

I love a long, hot shower at home, but here it was all wrong. The numbness of my forehead and scalp was disorienting. I couldn't tell when my head was fully beneath the stream of water, and I was too weak to turn around and look. In a few places with faint sensation, the water didn't feel wet or even warm; it was just pressure, which, aside from feeling strange, made me nervous. I imagined the droplets hammering into my scar, loosening the stitches, and my head filling with water like a fish bowl.

I tried to do things myself. I squirted some shampoo into my palm and felt around on the top of my head for where to shampoo. There were clumps of blood in my hair. My arms ached and I let my mom finish the job. I wanted to shave my armpits and wondered if now I'd always have to twist my neck around, as far as it could go, in order to see the left one.

The heat in there was beginning to be too much. I felt sleepy and nauseated. My mother quickly scrubbed my back and did some work on the glue that still clung to my arms and torso from a month's worth of IV tape and electrodes. Then she wrapped me in a combination of johnnies and towels, wheeled me back to my room, and got me dressed. She combed through my hair, picking out wet flakes of blood as she went. Then she rearranged my shoes along the far wall, straightened the soda water bottles on the windowsill, lined up the tissues, the call button, the hand sanitizer, and the can of ginger ale on my rolling bedside table, and left.

Crispy Rice and Eggs

Crispy rice and eggs was at the top of the breakfast list I made that day at Fletcher Allen. The recipe is a plan of action for any rice you may have left from the previous night's dinner. I usually add whatever other leftovers I find lurking in the fridge: sautéed greens, roasted carrots or brussels sprouts, chickpeas, anything that looks as though it would be at home on a bed of crisp rice beneath a runny fried egg. I eat my rice and eggs with hot sauce and a big spoonful of tangy yogurt on the side of the plate.

Olive oil

½ cup cooked brown rice (Go ahead and use white if that's what you've got.)

2 large eggs

Diamond Crystal kosher salt and black pepper

Plain, whole milk yogurt and hot sauce for serving, if you'd like

Pour a generous slick of olive oil into an 8- or 9-inch cast-iron pan and place over medium-high heat for 3 minutes. Scoop the rice into the hot pan and spread evenly across the surface with a spoon or rubber spatula. Reduce the heat to medium and cook for 60 to 90 seconds. Do not stir. While the rice is frying, crack the eggs into a small glass.

In the center of the rice, dig two holes, each one a little larger than an egg yolk. Pour one egg into each hole—some of the whites will seep into the surrounding rice—and cook for 2 minutes. Still, don't stir. Season with a generous pinch of salt and a couple grinds of black pepper. Turn on the broiler, and slide the pan beneath it for 1 to 2 minutes, until the whites are set and the yolks are warm but still runny.

Shimmy the rice and eggs onto a plate, helping it along with a spatula, if necessary. The whole thing will transfer like a pancake. Top with a few shakes of hot sauce and a generous dollop of yogurt, if using, and serve immediately.

Serves 1.

CHAPTER 14

Everything Happens

The next morning I met the weekend therapist for my first physical therapy session. She was tall, thin, and strong looking, probably in her early forties, and wore a purple linen shirt with short sleeves that buttoned at the biceps. "I have that shirt," I said, after we'd introduced ourselves. I thought it was a perfectly normal thing to say, but she didn't respond. Instead:

"Can you tie on your sneakers by yourself?"

Maybe I'd said the wrong thing. I imagined this healthy woman lifting the shirt from her drawer that morning, quickly pulling it over her head, and shooting out the door. Suddenly, what I'd said about the shirt felt ridiculous, like saying to Roger Federer, "I play tennis, too."

The therapist told me that my first task was to get comfortable walking again. I had no neurological damage, but after a month in bed, my muscles had grown so weak that I'd shake when I tried to stand.

She started me on the edge of the bed, had me lift one knee to the palm of my hand, then the other, kick my right leg out in front of me, then my left. It was time to stand up. She buckled me into a harness, two loops of nylon rope, one on each leg, and a handle that dangled behind me for her to grab on to. This way, I could practice walking without leaning on someone or something, and the therapist could still catch me if I started to fall. I was a dog on a leash.

We made our way slowly to the rehab gym at the end of the hallway. Me in the lead, the therapist hanging on to me from behind, my father pushing a wheelchair, just in case. The hallway felt as wide as a football field and at least twice as long. All that space and nothing to reach for made me anxious. The blindness made things worse. When I'd see someone coming, I'd freeze. Everyone was moving so quickly, the therapists, the nurses. Nothing felt safe. Because of the depth perception issue, I didn't notice that the floor rose in a slight ramp where it met the main walkway to the lobby. I just felt my heels tip back. I couldn't figure out if the slant was real or in my head, and I had the urge to squat down and crawl.

At the gym I was allowed to sit for a minute. When my legs stopped shaking, we got to work. I stood up; I sat down. Stood up, sat down. The therapist had me put my arms out to the sides while standing and close my eyes. I immediately started to tip and felt the tug of the harness keep me upright. She asked if I could raise one foot just a little bit off the ground. I tried, but my foot stayed glued to the floor. I looked over at my dad, who was watching from the side, and I started to cry. The therapist waited silently for me to cool it. She didn't say anything one way or the other about how I was doing, not a word about how it would get easier, how I would get stronger, that this was temporary. I knew better, but I started to wonder if that was because I wouldn't, and it wasn't.

On Monday, I met Jeff, the physical therapist who'd be with me the rest of the week. He was just a few years older than me, with a ponytail and a face that was easy on the eyes. We started out with more of the same. I'd march the hallway and Jeff would urge me to pick up the pace. In the gym he'd have me lift one foot. I could do it now, if only for a few seconds. I would wobble; he would catch me.

"I'm terrible at this," I whispered.

"Yeah," he agreed. "But you know what you're really good at?" I shook my head, genuinely unable to think of what I could possibly be good at just then.

"Not dying," he said. I smiled. He had a point.

"Hey," he said, grinning, "would you like to go outside?"

I grabbed my sweatshirt and followed him out and around to the side of the building. I tried to look casual as the double doors automatically swung open and the fresh air rushed in. Outside on my own two feet felt different from outside in a wheelchair. It felt good.

Jeff said he wanted me to try walking on grass. From the edge of the asphalt parking lot, I slid one foot over onto the lawn and pressed, then stepped all the way onto the spongy ground. It was uneven in places. My one eye couldn't tell me where, so I moved slowly, feeling ahead with my toe the way you do when you're bumping around in the dark. A tree sneaked up on me from the left and I walked into a thin-fingered branch. "Ouch," I said, running my thumb across the scratch on my forehead. The branch had been right in my blind spot. Nervous, I moved forward, ducking my head as though an invisible beam were hanging from the sky.

I think it was my second day at the rehab center when a neuropsychologist came by. His job was to make sure that, cognitively, I was as together as everyone seemed to think. He gave me lists of things to remember, then had me do math problems before asking me to repeat the items back. There were also scenarios, narratives that would end with the question "What would you do?"

One was about a lake in the woods. I'm out walking alone, the doctor told me. There's no one for miles around. As I approach the lake, I notice that there's a dock, and at the very end of it sits a two-year-old child, all by himself. "What would you do?" the doctor asked me.

"I'd get help," I said.

I waited for the doctor to say something back or nod his head or make any sound at all. He didn't.

"I mean, I'd ask him what he was doing there," I stammered. "If he was alone. Where his parents were." Wait, was that right? Do two-year-olds even talk? Maybe he'd been kidnapped and his abductor had left him there.

"I guess I'd take him with me and try to find his parents," I offered. Unless his parents were the ones who had left him there in the first place, in which case, should I really be tracking them down? Wasn't it irresponsible to hand this kid over to people capable of such neglect? Then again, was it legal *not* to?

"Or, no—" I paused. "I'd wait with him. For ten minutes, maybe. See if anyone turned up. If not, I'd drive him to the nearest police station."

The doctor listened unmoving, expressionless. *This is part of it,* I told myself. *He's not supposed to approve or disapprove.* That, or I was brain damaged after all, and I'd just said something so horrifying that he was contemplating reporting me to social services. Great. So much for ever having a child of my own. I couldn't even handle an imaginary one.

I thought about revising my answer yet again, but the doctor was on to something else. He wanted me to tell him about the fall in the conference center gym that morning, and about everything that had followed. I recounted for him the story as I understood it: the ruptured aneurysm, the surgery to fix it, the compressed optic nerve, the surgery after that.

"And why do you think this happened?" he asked when I was done.

I paused. I didn't understand the question.

"Why do I think this happened?" I repeated. "You mean, like, the aneurysm?"

He didn't answer.

"Okay . . . Um, from what I understand, there was a weak blood vessel in my brain. Over time, the vessel wall stretched, forming an aneurysm. About a month ago, it popped." I assumed he was after biology, since what else could he be asking? We were both silent for a minute.

"But why?" he wanted to know. "*Why* do you think it happened?" He was doing his best not to lead me. I wondered again what he was asking.

I'd assumed he was testing me to make sure I'd heard everything Dr. Tranmer had said and that I had a full understanding of my condition. That my answer hadn't satisfied him made me think I had missed some crucial aspect of how a ruptured brain aneurysm works. Finally, I spoke up.

"I don't think I'm answering your question."

"Well, sometimes people who have been through a thing like this say that they know why it happened," he explained. "They believe it's because of something they did or because of some reason they can point to."

"Wha—? I . . . No. No, I don't believe that." I shook my head.

The doctor's question was a version of something I'd start

hearing a lot: "Everything happens for a reason." People said it to me all the time. I know they meant to comfort; the words that followed usually had something to do with the good to be found in everything, or my "path" and how the meaning of my illness would one day be clear. I'd feel my chest tighten every time and do my best not to roll my eyes.

Everything happens for a reason? I don't see it that way at all. To me, only the first part is clear: Everything happens. Then other things happen, and other things, still. Out of each of these moments, we make something. Any number of somethings, in fact.

What comes of our own actions becomes the "reason." It is no predestined thing. We may arrive where we are by way of a specific path—we can take just one at a time—but it's never the only one that could have led to our destination. Nor does a single event, even a string of them, point decisively to a single landing spot. There are infinite possible versions of our lives. Meaning is not what happens, but what we do with what happens when it does.

"I don't know why it happened," I said. "Um . . . do you?"

CHAPTER 15

Becoming Home

I moved from Seattle to Cambridge alone, a month and a half after our city hall marriage and less than two months before our wedding. It was Labor Day weekend, and my graduate program was starting. Eli would remain in Seattle, wrap things up with work, fly in for our wedding at the end of October, and stay. A moving truck would follow in early November with both of our apartments' worth of stuff.

All my belongings would be in a Seattle storage unit until then, except for a few basics I'd crammed into my suitcase: a dinner plate, a cereal bowl, a frying pan, a small pot, one fork, one knife, and a spoon. At the hardware store near the university I bought a bamboo cutting board, a drinking glass, and an oversized mug. For furniture, I had an air mattress. That was it.

Eli had flown across the country with me for the long weekend to help get me settled into the apartment we'd rented. We picked up our keys, made ice cubes, bought toilet paper, milk, and eggs. On Sunday we drove up to the North Shore to see, for the first time, the wedding site we'd chosen from afar. We made a morning of it, wandering through the rooms of the Stuart-style mansion at the top of Castle Hill, walking the grassy slopes that tumbled a half mile down to the ocean, and stopping for cider doughnuts, hot out of the fryer, at the nearby farm.

We were on our way back to the highway when we spotted an antique wooden bench by the side of the road. Behind it was more furniture, spilling out from a large gray barn. We looked at each other. Eli turned the car around and pulled into the gravel driveway.

Up close, the bench was more imposing than it had been from the moving car. It was six feet long and solid oak, stained a deep chestnut, with six square, sturdy legs that matched the armrests. Its straight back was paneled with vertical slats hugged by two horizontal beams, like a railroad track. Into the top beam, someone had scratched "Bird."

We thought the bench was perhaps an old church pew, but there were no kneelers or slots on the back for books. The seller told us that it likely once lived in a railway station, sometime around the turn of the twentieth century. A few feet from the bench stood a narrow wooden table painted rust red. Along the length of both sides hung two hinged flaps that, when raised, turned it into a perfectly respectable dining table, small and square. A half hour later, we were on our way again, having purchased both.

Deliverymen arrived in Cambridge with the furniture a few days later. They heaved the bench into place against a long wall opposite the kitchen and put the table—a full two feet shorter than the bench in length—down in front of it. I'd borrowed a green canvas camping chair from an aunt and uncle when I moved in, and I set it up on the other side of the table, facing the bench. Now, in addition to an air mattress, I had an office and a dining room in one.

My office was the bench side. I kept my laptop on the table and piled my books and notes beside me on the bench, where there was more than enough room. When I got hungry, I'd adjourn to the other side of the table and take my meals in the green camping chair.

Food was limited to what I could prepare stovetop in my small frying pan and even smaller saucepan. There was a lot of rice and soft-boiled eggs. Canned sardines with mustard on crackers. Stir-fries happened, my one small spoon pushing broccoli spears around the pan. I chopped salads of cucumber, tomato, lettuce, and parsley with my dinner knife and topped them with olive oil, salt, and a squeeze of lemon. Then, because my only bowl was often busy with leftover rice in the fridge, I'd eat directly from the board. (I still do this, by the way, even with a cupboard full of dishes nearby. A salad board, stacked with thick slabs of bread and a wedge of sharp cheddar, makes a handsome solo feast, and a romantic meal for two.)

I'd likely have eaten similarly—sparely, simply—those first weeks, even with every knife, bowl, and baking sheet on-site. I like to break in a kitchen slowly. Get a sense of where it's best to stand when spreading peanut butter on toast, and how long it takes for the water from the faucet to run cold. Soon comes a pot of something, oatmeal or soup. I learn where the garbage pail should live, the oils, salt, and spices. How wide and hot the flame burns when the dial says medium-low. The first quiet beats of a rhythm emerge. Routine enters on tiptoe. You cannot rush these things.

Meanwhile, there was a neighborhood to explore.

The best part about being in a new city is figuring out what's there to eat. When I moved to Jerusalem for a year at twenty-three, I paced the supermarket aisles every day for a week, inspecting the packaged snack foods, the milk sold in bags, the yogurts and cheeses arranged on the shelves by percentage of fat. I bought halvah by the pound on Fridays at the open-air *shuk* and shaved away at it every afternoon to eat with oranges and tea. I wasn't only stocking my kitchen; I was mapping out a version of home.

Mine and Eli's new apartment was on the western edge of Harvard Square, steps from the university, a five-minute walk from the T, and, if you cut through Radcliffe Yard, less than one block over from a street called Brattle. Down a ways on this street, in the heart of the square, was Cardullo's, a small grocery selling foods from all over the world. My cookies were there, the amaretti in red and white tins. Also, marmalades, spices, and teas. They stocked treats from my life in England: Dairy Milk chocolate bars, hazelnut wafers, and HobNobs, digestive biscuits made with oats. Around the bend and across the street was the Algiers Coffee House. There I discovered *mujadarrah*, a mound of tender, spiced lentils, rice, and deeply cara-melized onions surrounded by a moat of yogurt. Continue on in that direction and you'd arrive at L.A. Burdick, home to the richest hot chocolate (dark or milk, your choice), served in small, white, handle-less mugs. And right next door, in an old yellow house set back from the street, was my favorite spot of all: a bakery called Hi-Rise Bread Company.

I knew right away that I'd found someplace special. Heaped on the wooden countertop were craggy scones, filled brioches, cookies, quick breads, and quiches. Golden loaves lined the side wall. They had egg sandwiches for breakfast, and killer oatmeal topped with toasted pecans and dried cherries. But what really tipped me off to the greatness of this place was a single word, printed on the menu in line with the heartier breakfast fare: toast. It was no side dish here.

My order came out in a paper-lined basket, one thick slice of yeasted cornbread and another from their Huron loaf, baked with whole wheat flour and sprouted wheat berries. Toasting here wasn't a hasty pass through a heated oven, but a thorough browning of crust and crumb. The surface of the bread had gone crisp, sharp, even, along the edges, with enough moisture left inside to lend some chew. Nestled into one corner of the basket were a triangular wedge of European butter, the kind with the highest fat, and a small cup of the bakery's homemade preserves. This was toast as it is meant to be: its own thing, a main event.

I went back to Hi-Rise as often as I could afford. Lunch there was a cup of soup and a savory raisin pecan roll, its crust so delightfully hard that the only fitting verb to describe the action of eating it is "gnaw." Or, if I was feeling big-stomached enough to tackle it, I'd have a grilled sandwich of caramelized onions, sautéed mushrooms, mustard, and two kinds of cheese. More often than lunch, though, I stopped by in the late afternoons for a single, perfect almond macaroon.

The Hi-Rise almond macaroon is plump and squat, a round, rosy cookie with a whole almond pressed into its belly and dusted with powdered sugar. Squeeze, and the crisp outer crust sinks into the chewy center. Two days a week I was done with classes by 4:00 p.m. I'd take the roundabout way home, along Brattle, and stop in at Hi-Rise. If they hadn't sold out yet that day, I'd buy my macaroon. The person behind the counter would twist it up in a square of white wax paper. I'd tuck it into my tote, walk home, fix myself a mug of Earl Grey tea with milk, pull the green camping chair over to the empty side of the room by the window, put my feet up on the radiator, and eat.

The power of that almond flavor was as potent a trigger as ever. I felt the tug of homes past, New York, Ohio, cooling almond cakes, red amaretto cookie tins lost and found. All of this in a new place, on the cusp of a new life. This after-school snack was my first real ritual in Cambridge, a way of digging my heels into fresh terrain. Untwisting my macaroon from its paper, my tote bag slumped on the floor beside me, the scene felt new but also not, as though I were claiming something that was already mine. It was the feeling of a home becoming home.

I looked forward to bringing Eli to Hi-Rise, and the week after our wedding, I did. November was unseasonably warm that year. I wore a brown embroidered skirt, a muted yellow sweater, leather riding boots, and a wedding band. It was lunchtime. We ordered a sandwich to share, plus two tart lemonades, and found a table out-side on the cobblestones beneath a tree. The woman who took our order recognized me. She knew we'd just married, that this was Eli, who was now here to stay, and with our order she brought a basket stuffed with treats to celebrate it all. Vanilla bean pound cake and a banana bread "cork," a brioche filled with apricot preserves, a homemade Oreo, and an almond macaroon for me.

My first few days in rehab, Eli was back in Cambridge. He'd gone home to get stuff in order, to catch up on work, and for a break. In addition to the feather pillow and purple fleece blanket I'd asked him to bring when he returned, I wanted one more thing: a Hi-Rise almond macaroon. I needed it, to know that my life back home actually existed, that I hadn't just dreamed it all up. It was real. Sometimes, during those long days and nights in Vermont, I had to convince myself that it was.

I sat in my pajamas in a chair by the bed and stuck my nose into the white paper bag. The macaroon smelled sweet and floral, as ever, and I couldn't wait to take a bite. But anesthesia does a number on your taste buds. The sweetness registered like something metallic. My tongue felt coated in fuzz. I dropped the other half back into the bag and told Eli to take it away.

Hi-Rise Almond Macaroons

When I asked René Becker of Hi-Rise Bread Company if he would share his almond macaroon recipe for this book, I had no idea that his own father had died of a ruptured brain aneurysm more than three decades ago. René's father experienced symptoms for years before finally seeing a doctor. By then, the aneurysm had grown too large to repair in surgery. He died four months later, when the aneurysm burst. René's recipe appears here in memory of his father.

For this recipe, you'll want to get your hands on Solo brand almond paste. Other popular brands are higher in sugar, which causes the macaroons to spread in the oven. With Solo, your macaroons will turn out nice and plump, just like René's.

One more thing: An oven thermometer is especially important when you're baking at a low temperature. Even ovens that are spot-on at higher temperatures can struggle to hit the mark at 300 degrees. Trust the thermometer and adjust the temperature accordingly.

1 pound Solo brand almond paste
1½ cups (300 grams) granulated sugar
¾ cup (90 grams) confectioners' sugar
⅛ teaspoon almond extract
3 large egg whites
About 30 whole almonds
Confectioners' sugar for dusting

In the bowl of a stand mixer fitted with the paddle attachment, mix the almond paste, sugars, and almond extract on low for 2 to 3 minutes, to form a crumbly, pebbly mixture. The largest almond paste pieces should be the size of small chickpeas. Add the egg whites and mix on medium-low for 3 minutes, pausing once to scrape down the sides of the bowl. Cover the bowl tightly with plastic and refrigerate overnight.

Preheat the oven to 300 degrees and line a baking sheet with parchment paper. Using 2 level tablespoons per macaroon, scoop the dough onto the prepared baking sheet, 1 to 2 inches apart. A cookie scoop comes in handy here because the dough is sticky. (I use a 1½-tablespoon scoop because it's all I have and it's close enough.) If you're using a measuring spoon instead of a cookie scoop, roll the dough into balls between your palms before placing them on the baking sheet. Press one almond into the top of each macaroon, and sift a generous amount of confectioners' sugar over top. Return the remaining dough to the fridge until you're ready to scoop the next round.

Bake for 28 to 33 minutes, rotating the baking sheet halfway through, until the macaroons are rosy on top and lightly brown on the bottom. Slide the parchment paper with the cookies onto a rack and cool completely. Repeat with the remaining dough, making sure to begin with a room temperature baking sheet.

Makes about 30 cookies.

CHAPTER 16

The Most We Could Do

I checked out of rehab in late September. I'd missed the season between summer and fall that feels like neither and both. Just skipped right over it, like an arm on a record player that lifts up from its groove, travels a few rings toward the center, and touches silently back down.

Eli was with me, and the walk to our car felt familiar and sweet. We might as well have been coming out of the movies or the grocery store. *I love this*, I caught myself thinking. Walking to the car was great.

I heard the keys scrape together in Eli's pocket when he reached for them and the beat of silence before he pressed the button on the fob. The locks thumped open like four tiny fist pumps and I felt the sound in my chest. I popped the handle on the passenger-side door, lowered myself onto the seat, and snapped the seat belt into its buckle. *Amen.*

Eli slammed my door shut and drove us out of there.

* * *

An hour south of Burlington, my friend Julia called. She and her husband, Eitan, were coming over with dinner that night, and she wanted to firm up plans and find out what else they could bring.

"Tell me what you want," she instructed. "You need to have exactly what you want." I told her which yogurt, which olives, which bread, but Julia would have gotten it right on her own.

Julia is a political fund-raiser who knows how to get things done. She's intuitive about what matters and what doesn't, which makes her decisive and quick, exactly the person you want planning your event for hundreds, or on the other end of the phone to advise you on anything. Julia has the best taste. Plus a keen understanding *of* taste. She once gave me a scarf, just because, that was unlike anything she'd ever seen me wear. It was perfect of course, just as she knew it would be.

Julia calls Eitan "homie." He's tall and thin, like Julia, but while she has olive skin and long black hair, he's rosy and fair, with blond hair and blue eyes. Eitan is easygoing, but no slouch. He was a PhD candidate in political science at Harvard when we met, and is the most efficient worker I know. He is also a total goofball. Once, in a debate with friends over the commonly accepted name for chocolate sprinkles—or would that be jimmies?—Eitan contended that an ice cream server would know what you meant no matter what you called them. He then marched up to the counter and, with a straight face, ordered a scoop of ice cream with "chocolate yum-yums, please." The server went right for those yum-yums. She didn't blink.

It's funny to think that we had met these two only eight months before I got sick, because they already felt like old friends. They had turned up in Cambridge the previous fall and we'd invited them to our Chanukah party. Eitan helped himself to a second plate of latkes while Julia proclaimed her love of sour cream. We liked them right away. They joined us for dinner one night not long after that, then we went to their place, and pretty soon we had an unspoken date almost every Friday evening at their table or ours.

Our friends Jonathan and Hila, who lived downstairs from Eitan and Julia, would join us, too. Jonathan was a fellow graduate student studying ancient Judaism and Christianity, warm and soft-spoken, and an intuitive cook. His wife, Hila, is Israeli, with a deep voice and a heart as big and fierce as they come. She was teaching second grade when we met, marveling daily at the American obsession with anti-bacterial hand sanitizer.

Potlucks make me nervous at best (lasagna with a side of pasta salad, anyone?), but with this crowd, they worked. Jonathan was our bread man, and I was in charge of dessert, and we juggled around the tasks of main dish, salad, and sides. These were three-, four-, five-hour meals, the kind where stories of rogue eBay sellers, and landlady drama, and impressions of professors and colleagues began all at once over soup, then stopped, started, and stretched through to the very last bites. There was always plenty of wine.

I hung up the phone. I wanted to go back to that table. I wanted things to be exactly as they had been. That feeling of forgetting yourself when you're swept up in conversation, joking and eating with friends, of being entirely at ease. It felt impossible now. I would miss things because of my eye. I was clumsy and slow. What if I felt that way forever? Eli cupped his hand around my knee.

"It's going to be okay," he said, reading my mind.

I put my hand on his. "Say more, say better." This was Eli's high school Talmud teacher's line after a student's first stab at explaining a difficult passage. We said it to each other all the time.

"Dr. Tranmer said six to eight months until you'll feel like your-self again. It sounds like a long time, but it's not. We just have to make it through the winter."

When he put it that way, it didn't sound so bad at all.

Eli unlocked our front door and I walked in. It smelled exactly right. Like us, though I hadn't been there in a month. It was late after-noon, my favorite time of day to come home. Orange light spilled through the south-facing windows onto the hardwood floor. I felt shy but welcome, as though I'd shown up late somewhere important to find that someone had saved me a seat.

This was the same apartment we had moved into that fall al-most three years earlier. I stepped from the doorway into the long main room. We'd set up the near end as our living room, our hand-some wooden bench opposite the green, down-stuffed sofa that I'd bought secondhand in Seattle. Over by the windows, on the other side of the fireplace, was our dining area. There stood our square, rust-colored antique table, and four wooden chairs that had been a craigslist find, one red, one lavender, and two pale green. I'd intended to paint them over in a single color when I bought them for my first apartment, but I'd never gotten around to it, and on second thought, I liked them the way they were. The bedroom was off to the right. I peeked in, eyed our blue and white quilt, and imagined myself slip-ping between the covers. I was glad for a bed to be just a bed again, and not a home base. I would sleep there at night and make it up in the mornings. During the day, if I had to lie down or sit, I'd do it somewhere—anywhere—else.

Our small, yellow-tiled bathroom was still small and yellow-tiled, and my little office was just as I had left it. A stack of books on deck for exam prep, a pack of sticky tabs, the yellow highlighter on its last legs that I needed to replace. My notebook was open to the to-do list I'd made up the night before I'd left for the conference. *Catherine the Great article. Revolution stuff. Fellowship paperwork. Revised reading lists to R. W. and J. H.* I'd written the call numbers of the next round of library books I needed on Post-it notes and stuck them along the bottom of my computer monitor. One had fallen onto the keyboard. I picked it up and flipped it over but didn't stick it back on.

Through the main room to the left was the large space intended as a dining room that we used instead as Eli's office and the catchall for an assortment of overflow dining and living room things. The enormous combination desk-bookshelf-filing-cabinet that Eli had built in his Seattle woodshop staked out the office side of the room. A long, narrow sideboard held our ceramic serving bowls and platters. And a sofa, a hand-me-down from Eli's parents, sat beneath the windows. The room made no sense.

So annoying, I thought, as always, shaking my head but smiling. Eli came up behind me. "You hate this room."

I turned to face him. "I really do."

He looped his arms around my waist and I rested my elbows on his shoulders.

"Hey, lady," he whispered.

"Hey."

I gestured with my head to the kitchen behind me.

"Would you go in there with me?" I asked. "I want to make a cup of tea." The words came out like a proclamation. *I hereby assert that I, Jessica Kate Fechtor, shall make a cup of tea!* Eli followed me in.

Our kitchen was a mere cubicle, tacked on to the hip of the dining-room-turned-office like a sidecar. The floor space measured thirty-five square feet, with just a small stretch of counter between the sink and the wall. The rest of the apartment had been preserved, more or less, in its original, early-twentieth-century design. Hardwood floors, high ceilings, a tiled working fireplace. There was even an old wall safe in the bedroom.

The kitchen, though, had been renovated and it no longer fit in. The cabinetry was made of cheap wood, in the style of bachelor-pad kitchens for the newly divorced. The cupboard doors were clunky with oddly rounded corners. Anything natural looking about the wood had been buffed out and stained over in a "honey color," you might generously call it, though really it was a dull tan. The counter was beige Formica and absorbed stains, and the floor was a grayish white linoleum that never looked clean.

But the oven had a gas range. It was old with worn dials and kept its heat beautifully, and glory be, there was a dishwasher. A garbage disposal, too. *This kitchen is a workhorse*, I decided when we first moved in. We just had to figure out how to make it so.

We started by rolling a small wooden cart against the back wall, trading a couple square feet of floor for a postage stamp of additional counter space. I did all my chopping there, and ingredient measuring, and mixing by hand. Eli installed a single shelf for spices on the wall above the cart and, from the ceiling overhead, he hung a pot rack. He'd found the studs in the ceiling and tested their strength by hanging from them in his climbing harness. "Hey, Jess!" he'd called across the apartment, and I'd walked in to find him dangling there, grinning. I gave him a gentle push, and when he swung back, he wrapped his legs around my torso, and I craned my neck upward and kissed his chin.

The refrigerator filled an odd little closet that led to the emergency stairwell. Or almost filled it. Shoved a few inches over, the fridge left us enough room to mount some shelves and baskets on the wall, and just like that, we had a pantry.

As renters, these things were the most we could do, but it was exactly enough.

We kept nothing in that kitchen that we didn't need, a pleasant side effect of which being that everything we had was both useful and used. There is a special kind of satisfaction in owning but three mixing bowls, a single favorite wooden spatula, and one each of the few pots and pans you actually like to cook in. You always get to use the spoon that feels best in your hand when that's the only one you've got. Our kitchen was kosher, so we had each of these things times two (one for dairy, one for meat), but even then, it all felt beautifully contained.

Peek in on a typical Friday afternoon, and you'd see everything in action: the floury top of the wooden cart where I shaped the challah dough; the stand mixer on the counter with its head reared back and cake batter dripping into the bowl; a pot of soup, nearly done, on the front right burner. All of these things happening not quite at once but in overlapping succession, baked, cooked, and spit out onto the sideboard in the "office" to cool.

This Friday afternoon was different. I'd make tea.

I opened up the cupboard and reached for the handle of a large blue and white mug, but when I closed my hand, I grasped only air. *Damn depth perception.* In a swift, fluid motion perfectly aligned with his target, Eli reached for the mug I'd just missed. I swatted at his arm and missed that, too.

"Don't help me."

I pressed in closer to the counter and focused my gaze on the mug. I was afraid I'd knock one of its neighbors to the ground, so I moved my hand slowly, as though casting a spell, until my fingertip bumped its rim. With the handle of the mug securely in my fist, I turned the knob on the sink and practiced finding the stream of cold water with my empty hand. Every time I went back in, the water met my fingers a fraction of a second sooner or later than I expected, based on what my eyes, no, my *eye*, was telling me. I tried to fill the mug, but I misjudged the distance and I clunked it into the faucet instead, which knocked it out of my hand. The mug dropped into the sink, and when I reached to grab it, my knuckles struck the bottom of the basin, too close, too soon.

Eli was standing on my left side, my blind side, but I could feel him looking at me. He picked up the mug and filled it with water, and I let him. I needed to sit down. Eli helped me to the sofa in his office by the window and I stretched out my legs along the cushions.

"Lady—" he started.

"Tell me what you're thinking," I demanded. I was afraid it was something horrible, that this wasn't what he'd signed up for, that he didn't think things would ever be normal again. Eli sat down on the sofa by my feet.

"I'm thinking about one day in the future when your brain has sorted things out and your eye is no longer an issue. When we don't even talk about it because you don't think about it."

I bit my lip and stared out the window. The sun was a splinter of fire above the trees. "Do you really believe that will happen?" I asked.

"Yes."

I comforted myself with the thought that Eli is usually right.

CHAPTER 17

Badass

Eitan and Julia arrived soon after dark. I'd moved to the sofa in the living room by the front door, and when Eli went down to let them in and help bring up the food, I practiced appearing normal. I sat up as straight as I could and relaxed my shoulders. I crossed and uncrossed my legs. I wanted to look like myself for my friends.

They were coming down the hallway now. I could hear Eitan laughing. I took a deep breath, raised my eyebrows, and tried on a big smile. Then I saw them, and with a jolt of adrenaline the smile turned real. My body instinctively jumped up to greet them, only the "jump" came out more like a slow-motion stagger.

"Hey!" Eitan shouted. He was wheeling one of those collapsible luggage carts, piled high with a vat of chicken soup, challah, and wine. Julia was right behind him carrying a roasted chicken.

"Jess . . . " she sighed. "I'm putting this in the kitchen. Homie," she said to Eitan, "homie, stop, you'll spill the soup. Unpack it right here."

"Oh, you guys, thank you so much," I said. "And hi!" I couldn't stop smiling.

"You look great, Jess. How do you feel?" Julia asked, still holding the chicken.

"Very happy to see you," I said.

She smiled back, her eyes wide, and shook her head. "Hold on, let me put this down."

Eitan stretched out his arms, then hesitated. "Uh, can I?"

"Yes, yes!" I said, but when I went in for the hug, he just barely laid his hands on my back, as if I were a mannequin whose limbs might fall out of their sockets. "I won't break." I laughed. So he squeezed, but only a little.

"They didn't shave your head. I can't even see your scar." Eitan was right. Dr. Tranmer had shaved only the slimmest line of hair before he'd made the incision. It was still a bit sore, and it itched a lot, and where the nerves had been cut my head felt tingly and numb, but even I had to admit when I saw myself in the mirror that it didn't look half bad.

"Oh, it's there," I promised him. "Here." I sat back down on the sofa and felt for the bumpy strip of scalp that ran from temple to temple an inch behind my hairline. Eitan bent down for a closer look.

"Holy shit," he said. "You are a total badass."

I liked that. I *was* badass.

Julia and Eli were getting things together in the kitchen.

"El, can I use this knife? I'm making the salad." Julia was all business as usual, and it was the best thing in the world. My friends were here! And if Julia was Julia, and Eitan was Eitan, then maybe I was, in fact, me. We all sat down together around the table. Eli blessed the wine and the challah, Eitan ladled soup into bowls, and Julia tossed the salad. Meanwhile, I sat, just sat, a guest at my own table yet unmistakably home.

Julia fretted about the chicken. She always does. About how it's never as good as her mother's, despite following precisely the same recipe. Julia's mother does, indeed, make a terrific chicken, but Julia does, too. I've told her that one million times, over every bird of hers we've ever eaten. I was thrilled that I'd almost died and still Julia said it, and we got to have that talk again. It was a welcome sign of normalcy. To care again about cooked chicken meant that the coast was clear.

Being sick is supposed to come along with grand realizations about What Really Matters, but I don't know. I think deep down, we're already aware of what's important and what's not. Which isn't to say that we always live our lives accordingly. We snap at our spouses and curse the traffic and miss the buds pushing up from the ground. But we know. We just forget to know sometimes.

Near-death forces us to remember. It pushes us into a state of aggressive gratitude that throws what's big and what's small into the sharpest relief. It's awfully hard to worry about the puddle of milk when you're just glad to be here to spill it.

Aggressive gratitude, though, is no way to live. It's too easy. We're meant to work at these things. To strive to know. Our task is to seek out what's essential, get distracted by the fluff, and *still* know, feel annoyed by annoyances, and find our way back. The so-called small stuff actually matters very much. It's what we push against on our way to figuring out how we wish to think and to be. We need that dialectic, and illness snatches it away. A stubbed toe, a too-long line at the post office, these things and the fluster they bring are signifiers of a healthy life, and I craved them.

At the end of the meal, Julia started to clear. I watched the way she pushed herself back from the table and floated effortlessly up from her chair, a plate in each hand. It looked like a dance to me. I wondered what it would take for me to move that way again. What was stopping me, exactly? There was weakness, for sure. My muscles were still remembering how to behave. I was sometimes nauseated and very, very tired. Plus this vision thing was so weird. The half-darkness, the tip of my own nose that I could see now all the time, the distrust of where things were in space, and thus, of where exactly I stood. I felt hemmed into my body, and at the same time, far removed. Yet there I was, sipping soup and talking chicken with our friends a month after I was, statistically speaking, supposed to be dead. Anything was possible.

Roasted Chicken

In *The Zuni Café Cookbook*, Judy Rodgers tells you everything you need to know about how to roast a chicken: Start with a small bird so that it will cook quickly and evenly. Dry it well, salt it early, and roast at high heat. No trussing—you want as much skin as possible exposed in the hot oven—and no rubbing down with butter or oil. In return, you get the perfect roasted chicken, juicy throughout with crisp, golden skin.

A word about salting: Rodgers advises "salting early," one to three days before cooking, to tenderize and flavor the meat. Kosher chickens have already been salted and have thus already reaped the tenderizing benefits of salting early, but for flavor, I season it with a bit more salt, as indicated below. A kosher bird still benefits from sitting a day or two uncovered in the fridge. The skin will turn out especially crisp. I serve this chicken with crusty bread and a simple salad.

For the chicken:

    1 3- to 4-pound chicken, giblets removed
    4 sprigs fresh thyme, rosemary, or sage

¾ teaspoon Diamond Crystal kosher salt per pound of chicken
(¼ teaspoon per pound if you're using a kosher chicken)
About ¼ teaspoon freshly ground black pepper

Pat the chicken very dry, inside and out, with paper towels. Slip a finger beneath the skin on each breast near the edge of the cavity to form a couple of pockets, then do the same on the thickest part of each thigh. Slide an herb sprig into each of the four pockets.

Season all over with the suggested amount of salt and black pepper, and sprinkle a bit of each just inside the cavity. Refrigerate, uncovered, for 24 to 48 hours. Remove from the fridge half an hour prior to roasting, and give it another few pats with a paper towel to get rid of any excess moisture.

Preheat the oven to 475 degrees.

Place a 10-inch cast-iron or stainless steel skillet over medium heat for 4 minutes. Set the chicken breast-side up in the pan. You should hear it sizzle. Transfer the pan to the oven. If the skin doesn't begin browning within 20 minutes, raise the temperature to 500 degrees until it does. If, on the other hand, the skin begins to blacken or smoke (blistering is fine and welcome), lower the temperature to 450 degrees.

After about 30 minutes, turn the bird over and roast for another 15 to 20 minutes, then flip one last time and roast breast-side up for another 5 to 10 minutes to recrisp the skin. The chicken is done when a thermometer inserted into the hip meat (between the leg and the breast) reads 165 degrees. Transfer the bird to a large plate or carving board, and let rest for 15 minutes before cutting it into pieces.

Serves 3 to 4.

CHAPTER 18

A Certain Kind of Best

I'd been promoted. For weeks I'd been a professional sick person. Now I was a professional recovering person. In some ways, it was a lateral move. I still slept a lot, stayed mostly indoors, and ate food that other people prepared, but I appreciated the new title. Plus, there were perks. My own bed, for example, and a dresser full of clothes.

Before I was discharged from the hospital, a nurse, or maybe a social worker, had come to talk to me about this mysterious thing called recovery. Even after rehab, she explained, there would be a ways to go.

"Each day, you'll be able to do one thing, and it will totally wipe you out. That might be the case for a while."

"What do you mean by 'one thing'?" I wanted to know. I envisioned a trip to the grocery store or baking a cake.

"That's hard to say," she said. "It might mean a phone call with a friend. A shower."

Not possible, I thought. But she was right. In fact, forget a shower, an event which to me includes washing my face, scrubbing my body, shampooing and conditioning my hair, plus, because I do some of my best thinking in there, a few minutes of standing around. A shower means all of these things. When I first got home, though, I'd get in and have to choose. I could wash my hair *or* my body, not both, before exhaustion sneaked up and kicked me behind the knees. I'd call through the wide-open bathroom door to Eli, who'd wrap me in a towel and help me to the bed, where I'd sit with my heart pounding, sipping cranberry juice until the waves of nausea passed. Then I'd need a nap. This "one thing" thing was no joke. Apparently a healing brain takes its sweet time. A physical therapist came a couple of times my first week home and we practiced climbing stairs. That counted as a thing and a half, at least, as did a visit from a friend.

If I was feeling physically better each day, I couldn't tell. I was wiped out. Sometimes my body ached, like at the beginning of a flu. That was new. No wonder, though, I figured. Recovery was hard work.

"You know what?" I said to Eli one morning. "It's okay that this happened to me."

"Is that so?" he said.

What I meant was that I felt—I was suddenly quite sure—that I could handle this. That my life could handle it. An energizing gratitude crept into my bones.

"Does my face look swollen to you?" I asked Eli. I was standing in front of the mirror in our bedroom.

"Does your face look swollen?" Eli has a way of repeating a question before he responds.

"I asked you first," I said. "I mean, more swollen. Differently swollen."

He looked at me. "Nope."

I wasn't so sure. I'd been home for a week, and I thought my left eye looked strangely, I don't know, buglike. Only sometimes, though. On and off. A lot of the time my eye looked normal. Or maybe all of the time it looked normal, and I was imagining things. Probably.

"You can call Dr. Tranmer if you're concerned." Eli obviously wasn't.

"Yeah, okay. Maybe."

Before I had a chance to, Dr. Tranmer called me to check in. I mentioned the bulging eye and the body aches that came and went.

"A little bit of swelling is still normal this far out," he assured me. "But otherwise you should be feeling pretty darn great."

I wasn't.

My father arrived from Ohio late that afternoon with my youngest sister, Anna. Half sister, technically, but we've never emphasized the half. I have a half brother, too, named Caleb. My stepmom, Amy, is their mom and we share a dad. My younger sister, Kasey, and I share a mom *and* a dad. In descending birth order it's me, Kasey, Caleb, and Anna, and now you know the whole family.

Anyway, Anna. She was fourteen then, and through the hospital system she'd sent me e-mails bursting with exclamation points and all the latest very important news about her classes and the JV tennis team. "I know that you have been hearing nothing but stuff about your brain, so I'm gonna try to keep it as non-brainy as possible," she wrote, which was excellent. She hadn't seen me yet.

I opened the front door myself when they arrived. I was wearing the new clothes my mother had picked up for me in Burlington—jeans one size down that actually fit and a short-sleeved, dark green turtleneck with three buttons along the collar and pleats across the chest. I caught a glimpse of Anna's wide eyes and nervous smile in the doorway, then watched relief register and her face relax. *Good,* I thought, *I must look okay.*

Anna, Eli, and I sat down on the green sofa and my dad placed a cardboard box on the coffee table in front of us.

"Mom made you these," Anna said as I folded open the top flaps. Chocolate chip cookies. Eli took one bite and said, "Toll House." He'd called it right: the recipe from the back of the yellow chocolate chip bag. Toll House cookies are chewy and flat, faintly rippled like unsmoothed bedsheets, with a sugary crumb and those unmistakable Toll House "morsels." I recognized them, too. They were the only chocolate chip cookies I had ever baked. That's because they were, in my mind, a certain kind of best. Not "best" as in the best in the world, or even the best I'd ever eaten, but "best" in the sense that I'd choose them, at least some of the time, over ones that actually are. They were "best" because they meant something to me.

I made Toll House cookies for the first time when I was eleven years old, with Amy. My sister Kasey and I had met Amy a couple of years earlier, in 1989, at a Dairy Queen in Cleveland. (It is a wise man who stages his daughters' initial encounter with his soon-to-be fiancée over ice cream.) She wore silver howling-at-the-moon coyote earrings and ordered a Blizzard. I liked her, which was good, because in 1991, she married my dad.

They moved into an old house in Cleveland Heights, and that was where the cookie making began. Amy had a wide-mouthed yellow plastic pitcher, and we'd mix the dough in there by hand with a wooden spoon. I'd never used a wooden spoon before. My mother called them unsanitary, but I thought it was beautiful, and soft and warm, besides. Cookie making became kind of our thing, Amy's and mine. I liked that we had a thing.

I had baked with my own mother as a kid, but this was something new. My mother and I made sugar cookies, cupcakes, and brownies galore mainly as projects, fun things to do together that might have been replaced by any number of other fun things. Baking was special because it wasn't part of our everyday. When we pulled out the mixing bowl and electric beaters, it was an occasion. With Amy, it was different. She baked all the time, whether I was around or not. When we baked together, she was sharing with me this thing that she did and loved. She was letting me in, and I her. We were becoming a family.

At some point that weekend it was just Anna and me, and I asked her how things were at home. She told me how nuts it had been with Dad and her mom flying back and forth, how they were so annoying, always talking about me and the surgery, so stressed out, crying.

"They made such a big deal out of it," she said, rolling her eyes. "I mean, it's not like you were going to die or anything."

I appreciated the vote of confidence.

Whole Wheat Chocolate Chip Cookies

While I will never turn down a Toll House cookie, a new chocolate chip cookie came into my life a few years back that instantly became my go-to. The cookie's defining feature is that it's made exclusively with whole wheat flour. That sounds annoyingly virtuous for a chocolate chip cookie, but the whole wheat's not there to be healthy. It's there because it tastes good. When I first discovered these cookies, I baked them for everyone I knew. My friends all had a guess about what was different in these cookies, but very few called out the whole wheat flour. They asked instead if I'd put ground walnuts in there, or oats, or an earthy spice of some kind. One person insisted I'd browned the butter. Nope. It was just the whole wheat talking.

These cookies bake up fat, with a crisp, crustlike exterior. On the inside, they're soft, even borderline flakey. The genius behind them is Kim Boyce, who published the recipe in her cookbook, *Good to the Grain*. Her specialty is taking whole grains, figuring out their particular powers of flavor and texture, and harnessing them in the service of baked goods that are astoundingly delicious. (If you ever visit her Bakeshop in Portland, Oregon, please have one of everything for me.)

The only thing better than a Kim Boyce chocolate chip cookie is a Kim Boyce chocolate chip cookie made from dough that's been aged for a day or two. I like to prepare the dough, scoop it into individual cookies, and store them in the fridge on a baking sheet wrapped in plastic. Then, when the mood strikes, I bake them off, a cookie or two at a time.

3 cups (340 grams) whole wheat flour

1½ teaspoons baking powder

1 teaspoon baking soda

1 teaspoon fine sea salt

1 cup (2 sticks; 226 grams) unsalted butter, softened to cool
    room temperature and cut into ½-inch pieces

1 cup (200 grams) dark brown sugar

1 cup (200 grams) granulated sugar

2 large eggs

2 teaspoons pure vanilla extract

8 ounces (227 grams) bittersweet or semisweet chocolate (I use something in the 62–72 percent range), roughly chopped into ¼- and ½-inch pieces

Sea salt flakes, like Maldon

Line a baking sheet with parchment paper.

Whisk together the flour, baking powder, baking soda, and fine sea salt in a large bowl. Put the butter and sugars in the bowl of a stand mixer fitted with the paddle attachment, and mix on low speed until just blended. Scrape down the sides of the bowl with a spatula. Add the eggs one at a time, mixing well after each addition. Mix in the vanilla.

Add the flour mixture to the bowl, and blend on the lowest speed until the flour is just barely incorporated. Add the chopped chocolate, and mix with a rubber spatula. If there are any small pockets of flour lurking in the dough, rub them in with the spatula or your hands. (Better to leave off using the mixer at this point so that you don't overwork the dough.)

Scoop the dough, 3 level tablespoons per cookie, onto the prepared baking sheet. I use a 1½-tablespoon cookie scoop and pile one level scoop on top of another. You can crowd the mounds of dough shoulder to shoulder on the single sheet so that they won't take up too much room in the fridge. (You'll move the cookies to a separate sheet when you're ready to bake them.) Wrap the dough in plastic and chill for 24 to 48 hours.

When you're ready to bake, heat the oven to 350 degrees and line another baking sheet with parchment paper. Place 6 to 8 mounds of prescooped dough onto the prepared pan, leaving about 3 inches between each cookie. Press a few sea salt flakes into the top of each mound.

Bake for 16 to 20 minutes, rotating the sheet halfway through, until nicely brown but still soft. Slide the parchment paper with the cookies onto a rack and cool completely. Repeat with the remaining dough, making sure to begin with a room temperature baking sheet.

Makes about 20 cookies.

CHAPTER 19

Medium Dreadful

That Sunday, in the last hours of my dad and Anna's visit, a full-fledged fever came on and stayed. We called Dr. Tranmer, who said it sounded like I'd picked up a bug, and to feel better soon. I got into bed.

My head throbbed and the coming-and-going swelling thing I thought I'd noticed became the coming-and-going swelling thing I noticed for sure. Eli saw it now, too, but perhaps this was just what recovery looked like a few weeks out from brain surgery?

The next morning I felt no worse, and maybe even a little better. My fever returned to a low-grade something or other that was questionably a fever at all. Rosh Hashanah, the Jewish New Year, was beginning that night. Friends of ours knocked on our door to deliver a holiday meal.

Then things got bad fast. My fever spiked to 104 and wouldn't come down, and the swelling was no longer going. Instead, it was spreading; it was in my forehead and temple now, too. Eli folded me into the car with an ice pack for my head and we drove to the ER.

They brought me back right away, which didn't make me nervous but should have, and paged a neurosurgery resident. That got my attention.

"Why?" I asked Eli. "Why?" I was scared. "I'm afraid they're going to cut into my head again."

"That's not going to happen," he said. I knew it was improbable. I'd said my fear out loud in part not because I believed it could happen, but to make sure it didn't. Magical thinking: To say it was to ward it off.

The next hours and days get swimmy in my mind. I know that there was an MRI, and that soon after, I was admitted. My fever stayed high. My head continued to swell. None of the doctors knew for sure what was happening to me, but from what I understood it was one of two things: a cerebral spinal fluid leak or an infection. There was also a third option: both. A neurosurgery resident told me that they would operate, then a few hours later said that they wouldn't and disappeared.

Next came a trip to a neuro-ophthalmologist in the building next door. Someone carted me over in a wheelchair in my johnny with a blanket around my shoulders and one across my lap. I hadn't been allowed to eat or drink since I'd been admitted—was surgery a possibility still?—so I was hooked up to an IV. It rattled along beside me. The office was in the hospital, but regular people went there, fully clothed ones who'd walked or driven there alone. I sat in the waiting room right along with them while they read their magazines and tried not to look. I was too sick to care if they did.

"Oh no," the doctor said when he saw me. By now my face was contorted from the swelling. My left eye bulged and my temple was a giant pillow of a thing, yanking my cheek up with it; my skin stretched unnaturally across my forehead, a hard, protruding ridge. I was flushed and sweating from fever, and my Frankenstein scar peeked out from beneath my matted hair. I'm not sure what this doctor was looking for, but he must not have found it, because he sent me back to my room and I never saw him again.

I was doing that thing now that I'd practiced in Burlington when the pain had been at its worst. I pictured it not inside me, but right alongside, and shut myself down to increase the space between us. Sometime in the night, I had to use the bathroom. I pressed the red call button, as I'd been instructed, and an unsmiling nurse came to help me along. When I was through, I realized my gown was wet.

"It must have dropped into the toilet," I told her.

"It will dry," she said.

I got back into bed.

Morning again. A test. I lay on a table and someone strapped my ankles down. Slowly, the table tilted back, farther, farther, until I was hanging upside down. The pain and the pressure were too much and a roar, half scream, half sob, came barreling out of me. The doctors lowered me down and into the waiting scanner so they could snap their shot right away. "Almost there, almost there, almost there . . . Done," I heard one of them say. I strained to lift my head up from the table and green vomit shot out of my mouth. Then I lay there, sobbing and heaving, until someone wheeled me away.

An infection? A leak? They still didn't know. But yes, they would operate. They'd slice back in along my old incision, peel my forehead down once more, suck some fat from my belly to plug up the hole if there was one, and deal with the infection if that was what they found.

I didn't care. I just wanted them to fix it.

Waking up from surgery is rapture. Nurses and doctors will tell you that you won't remember it. Some people must not, but I always do.

I love the first breath, how it feels spiked with extra oxygen sneaked into the atmosphere when no one was looking, like rum in the punch bowl at a high school dance. Along with it comes the awareness that I'm alive and not dead, then the druggy realization that I have arms and legs and a body and there is no pain. I feel cured. A pleasant heaviness pins me to the gurney, and at the same time I'm so light, I think I might float away. Through the haze of anesthesia, the fluorescent bulbs are beautiful, the way they glow and light up the hospital corridor. I feel warm and safe, and I am only glad.

As far as I was concerned, the worst thing had happened— another surgery—and I had made it through. It, whatever "it" was, was over. Someone wheeled me from the recovery bay to my room and I waited for Eli to be allowed in so he could confirm what I already knew: that all was well and we were done and I'd be going home soon.

But something was off. I could tell when Eli walked in. He sat down on the bed and put his hand on my leg. Why did he look so sad?

"Jess . . ." he started. It was a voice I'd only ever heard once, five years earlier, when he'd called me from the other side of the world to tell me my grandmother had died. Was that what was going on? Was I dying? They must have found something when they went in. I studied his stricken face and waited for him to go on.

"You have an infection," he explained. "It got into your skull and a piece of it, the piece they sawed into when they fixed your aneurysm, was so diseased that they had to take it out and throw it away."

"Okay," I said, bracing myself for the part where he'd tell me I was dead.

"They scraped out as much of the infection as they could, and sewed you back up, but you have a deep indentation above your left eye where the forehead bone used to be. You'll be like this for a year, and then you'll have to have another surgery so they can fill in the hole. They're going to give you a helmet . . ." His voice trailed off.

"Okay," I said again, still waiting for the terrible news.

"They've started some strong antibiotics for the infection and you'll be on them for a while. At home, too. Through an IV."

Clearly I was missing something. "I don't understand. Will I be okay?"

"Yes." *Wait, what?* I didn't know if I wanted to kiss him or punch him.

"I'm so sorry, Jess—"

"Eli!" I was actually laughing. A helmet? Some drugs? Big deal! I asked for a mirror, too relieved to feel nervous. How bad could it be? And then I saw it. Part of my skull was missing, all right. My head looked like a partially deflated beach ball that someone had bashed in with his fist. The top of my left eyebrow disappeared into the hollow. There was no forehead above my unseeing eye.

"Okay . . ." I said. "Okay. Okay. But this is temporary, right? This is temporary." Eli nodded. I made him tell me a few more times that I'd be fine, just to be sure, then sent him to get my parents and sank back into the last delicious moments of my postanesthesia euphoria.

This time the surgeons had gone just sort of right up *to* the brain, without going inside, and there hadn't been a hemorrhage, so things were only a little bit dreadful—okay, medium dreadful—and only for a couple of days. But sometime in there, as soon as the anesthesia had fully lifted, I noticed something: I couldn't smell.

The antibacterial Cal Stat that everyone rubbed on their hands before they approached my bed, the trays of hospital food that went uneaten before someone carted them off, the sickly sweet scent that hung over the cans of vanilla Ensure, my mother's perfume, Eli's unshaven skin: nothing.

My surgeon surmised that with all of his scraping around in there, my olfactory nerves had been damaged. He said it casually, as though explaining what happens when you skin your knee.

"Will it come back?" I wanted to know.

"Probably not," he said lightly, and then, "But you don't really need your sense of smell anyway." I know he wasn't trying to be cruel. From a medical perspective, he must have meant, it doesn't matter whether or not you can smell. I was horrified.

Strangely enough, my father had lost his own sense of smell about ten years earlier in a Razor scooter accident. (Wear helmets, friends.) He discovered the deficit one morning not long after, when he splashed puddle after puddle of aftershave onto his face, finally determining that it must somehow have expired and lost its scent. When he walked downstairs and into the kitchen, my brother nearly keeled over.

There are some funny stories about toast left to burn, and the dog puke in the basement that once went unnoticed for days while Amy and the kids were away. He missed things, though. We'd forget sometimes and moan over the aroma of the brownies baking in the oven, then see my dad stick out his lip in an exaggerated pout. I remember a time one summer when my brother and sister ran in from the backyard. They were maybe seven and eight then, and he'd said to me, "You know what I miss? The smell of their sweaty little heads."

I thought of that now, of all the scents I'd miss, and all the scents I'd never know, and for the first time since my fall, I felt a tiny black hole stretch open inside of me. For the first time, the thought occurred to me that maybe everything was *not* going to be okay. An eye. My sense of smell. What was next?

But the fever was coming down, and soon it disappeared. The antibiotic was working. Someone came in to fit me with my helmet, which turned out to be a hockey helmet. An actual hockey helmet. White plastic, with a thick elastic chin strap secured on either side to a black rubber loop by each ear. It came down over the part of my face that was missing and, by hiding the defect, made me look sort of normal. As normal as a woman in a hospital gown and a hockey helmet can look, anyway. I had some soreness in my neck that my doctor told me was expected after an infection like that. My glands and lymph nodes were in overdrive, he said, but that would clear up soon. I could go home the following day.

Before I was discharged, an occupational therapist came to evaluate me. It's clear to me now that she was young—newly and thus faithfully wed to the protocols she'd learned in her training. She carried a clipboard with a list of questions.

"Do you live in a house or in an apartment?"

"An apartment."

"How did you get inside before you got sick?"

"Excuse me?" It was the "before you got sick" that threw me. The implication that I'd have to do it another way now.

"Are there stairs?"

"Yes, a few up to the front door."

"Is there an elevator inside?"

"Yes."

She scribbled some notes onto her pad.

"Did you toilet yourself before you got sick?" I couldn't believe she was serious.

"Yes."

"How did you bathe before you got sick?" The healthy, unterrified version of myself would have realized that all of this "before you got sick" business was just standard language. The therapist had probably been taught to ask the same things in exactly the same way of each of her patients, many of whom—unlike me—had limited mobility before whatever had landed them in the hospital, or had suffered debilitating physical or cognitive deficits. But hadn't she read my file? And if she had, and she still thought these questions applied, was I worse off than I knew? Panic crept up along the back of my neck.

"I got into the shower. I washed my hair." My throat was so tight that it hurt to talk. Why was I speaking in the past tense?

"Can you show me how?" she asked. I lifted both of my hands to my head and wiggled my fingers around. She scribbled another something down. Silent tears had begun to squeeze out from the corners of my eyes. I wiped at them with the back of my hand.

"Just another few questions. What did you like to do before you got sick?"

"I liked to cook?" I squeaked.

"Well," she said, "maybe we can get some peanut butter up here and you can spread it on some bread. Would you like that?"

"No!" I gasped. I was really crying now. "No, I would not like that!" Would that be the extent of my cooking now? "After," as opposed to "before"?

The therapist was assessing my ability to take care of myself, but that was the least of what I wanted to be able to do. I wanted to take care of *other* people. Host dinners at my table the way I'd always done. Chop the garlic, stir the soup, slice the cake. The cake I'd baked.

I went home. My mother was with us now. She had washed the

sheets and made up the bed, and I tried to sleep, but the pain in my neck was building. I ran my doctor's reassurance on a loop through my brain and breathed, and Eli hooked me up to the IV as he'd been shown. I watched the medicine drip into my body and drifted off.

The pain choked me awake, stabbing into my neck on both sides. It was dark now, near midnight, and I could tell that I had a fever. Eli stuck the thermometer under my tongue and we watched the numbers climb. I was back in the hospital that night.

This part was worse than anything that had happened so far. It feels crazy to say, after the hemorrhage and the surgeries, but it was. I couldn't take the whiplash, the you're-okay-you're-not-okay. Residents disagreed loudly over my bed about what was going on. Doctors said different things. The infection was raging, or it was on its way out, or the medicine was working, or it was time to try another, or my blood counts were off and I'd be put in isolation, but no, wait, my blood was fine and now they'd do an MRI. Someone wheeled me off downstairs and left me in the hallway, but no one came to get me, until a person finally stopped, and I heard him ask around to find out where I had to be. And still the fever, and the pain, so a nurse gave me a button and said push it for the morphine, and I did, but no relief, until finally, "We think you might be having a reaction. You're going off the vancomycin, and we're starting something new."

My fever rose and fell as the offending antibiotic made its way out of my system. I was afraid to be alone anymore in the hospital. Eli had come down with a cold and had to stay away for a while, so my mom and dad took turns spending the night in the reclining chair by my bed. On its way to breaking, the fever reached its peak. My vision blurred and I started to shake, and my mother called the nurse, who came with ice to cool me down. I was shivering so hard that my arms and legs were practically flailing. Without any sense of what I was doing, I writhed away from the ice. I didn't mean to. I didn't not.

The nurse was cross. "Are you refusing treatment?"

"That's not what's going on," I heard my mother say.

And then everything went white. *I need this to be over,* I thought. *I'm okay now to be dead. Be not awake now. Please. I can't. It's fine. I'm done.*

CHAPTER 20

Three Mushrooms

I came home in mid-October. There was no relief in it this time. No peeking into rooms or fumbled cups of tea. I don't even remember walking through the door. I needed to be lying down and went straight to bed.

It wasn't only that I was sicker than I'd been before the infection. This time, I was afraid. Without the round-the-clock monitoring and a surgeon on call I felt a constant tickle of panic. Bad things kept happening. Doctors had told me I was fine when I wasn't, again and again and again. Eli knew me better than anyone and even he hadn't seen that I wasn't okay. He'd said there would be no more surgery. He'd said we were done. When we weren't, the best doctors in the world had struggled to find out what was wrong, and then to treat it.

I'd try to talk myself down: *They sent me home from the hospital. That means I'm improving, right? That I'm going to be okay?* But I'd ended up right back there the last time. I'd heard what my infectious disease doctor had said right before I checked out: "You're not out of the woods yet."

On and on my thoughts unspooled. What was I to believe now, and whom? *No one,* my anxious brain answered. It was my job, then, and mine alone, to make sure that I stayed alive. I put myself on high alert. Everything was a symptom that pointed to a recurrence of infection, a stroke, a heart attack, the rupture of my residual aneurysm. I was a helmet-clad sentinel, half blind, unable to smell, with a busted-up skull and an itchy trigger finger. I had no idea what I was looking for, but I was ready to shoot at anything that moved.

I felt dizzy and nauseated. My vision blurred. A swimmy ache in my shoulders and chest would come and go along with a low-grade fever. I'd break out into a sweat while sitting perfectly still, sip at the air, trying and failing to top off my lungs enough to feel full. I took the sedatives the doctor had prescribed, but adrenaline fought back and won. I lay awake, pummeled by a sympathetic nervous system stuck in simultaneous fight and flight, and traced the indigo block-print flowers on the quilt with my thumbs.

The trips to the ER and back during the days that followed didn't help matters. There was a scare over my PICC line, the catheter for the antibiotic that ran through a vein in my arm to my heart; an intestinal infection (the dreaded C. *diff*); and a new, higher fever that we feared was something, but wasn't.

Pseudomonas, the bacteria that had exploded in the tissue surrounding my brain and taken out that chunk of skull, is insidious. It knows how to hide, get very quiet, make itself invisible, then flare back up in a flash. That was why I would have to wait a year for the reconstructive surgery, to be sure that the infection was truly gone and not lurking, undetected, in my healthy tissue and bone. It was why, three times a day, Eli plugged me into an antibiotic that, even as it drove out the infection, made me feel sicker. I lost more weight. My tongue turned black. My joints ached, and when I touched my head, strands of hair came off in my hand.

Two months earlier, mine had been the body of a healthy twenty-eight-year-old, fitter than ever before. It wasn't supposed to be capable of this kind of collapse. But it was, of course. A body always is. I was furious with myself for not seeing that, for ever thinking that health was something I could count on. I'd always had excellent luck and my genes were enviable. No broken bones, maybe one cold a year, great-grandmothers and great-great aunts who lived into their nineties. I took care of myself. I ate oatmeal and kale. I flossed. I followed the rules that were supposed to keep me safe.

Don't get me wrong—I'd imagined illness. Critical, devastating, out-of-nowhere illness. I was right there in the imagined hospital rooms of my worst nightmares, alongside Eli or a parent or a friend. Only I was never the one in the bed. I was the big-hearted helper, the devoted cheerleader. I brought the cookies.

Eli was in charge of the medical stuff. He kept track of my medications, and when it came time for my middle-of-the-night antibiotics, he would shut off his alarm and creep around to my side of the bed. By the time I would open my eyes, he'd be standing over me in his underwear, hooking up the plastic tubing to the port in my arm. I was quiet sometimes, and sometimes I'd cry. I remember him brushing the hair away from the missing part of my face and smiling down at me with crinkly eyes. He moved quickly, carefully. Then he'd shut out the lights and I'd float off into a foggy half sleep while the bag emptied into my body.

My mother stayed with us, on an air mattress in the living room, during my first few weeks home. It was important, she said, that Eli and I remain husband and wife through this, and not just caregiver and patient. She helped me with the most basic, private tasks, rubbing my feet with lotion, holding me upright on the toilet when my legs would start to shake. Sometimes, she would bathe me, wash and fold our laundry, prepare lunch, and then quietly slip out for an hour or so, leaving us to act out, as best we could, something resembling our normal life. Full garbage bags disappeared to the basement bins, beds got stripped and remade, dishes washed, counters wiped clean. My nightstand, a jumble of medicine bottles, hand sanitizer, tissues, juice glasses, and a thing I'd breathe into to exercise my lungs, got straightened and cleared. She didn't ask; she did.

When I was a little girl, my mother was everything to me. All the more so after my parents separated. I was seven, and they divorced a few years later. I thought the intervening time meant that in the end they might stay together, but it was actually just how these things sometimes go. In the years after my father left, my mother was finishing up her master's degree and working full-time as a management consultant, yet I never remember her not being around. She drove me to play rehearsals, talked me through all of my childhood stresses and woes, taught me how to visualize success the night before big tests, and read every word of every school paper I wrote until I went off to college. She was the most capable human being I could imagine.

So it scared me to sometimes find her in the middle of the night, weeping on her bathroom floor. She'd have her knees up under her nightgown and a roll of toilet paper in one hand. She'd tear off a few squares at a time to blow her nose. I'd do my seven- or eight- or nine-year-old best to comfort her, sink down beside her, wish that I could gather her up into my small body and keep her safe. When I would start to cry, she would gather *me* up, and I'd press my cheek into her chest wet with both of our tears. In the morning she'd be back to it, writing cheery notes in the pages of my notebook for me to find in the middle of my school day, flashing me a sign language "I love you" as I climbed onto the bus.

Most nights, we had dinner together the three of us, my mom, my sister Kasey, and me. While my mother mourned the loss of her marriage, she also mourned the loss of her family—of a certain *idea* of family that meant a mother and a father under one roof and forever-and-ever love. Family dinner was a way of shoring up what was left, of making our family feel like three out of three instead of a remainder. It was a sign that all had not been lost.

My mother wasn't the type to cook up a storm at the start of the week, planning and freezing and making lists. We had leftovers sometimes, sure, but most of the time she came home after work and started from scratch. She'd snap on the small television she kept on the kitchen counter and cook through the six o'clock news, *Wheel of Fortune*, and halfway through *Jeopardy*, at least. Then the TV would go off and we would sit down to eat, my mother at the head of the long antique table that she and my father had bought together years before, Kasey and I across from each other on either side.

Dinner was never a little of this, a little of that, but something hot that had a name. Baked Salmon (with lemon pepper and dill); Stir-Fry (with water chestnuts and baby corn). There was a casserole with elbow noodles, frozen vegetables, and ground meat that you spooned from a glass bowl; and—an exception to the hot rule—the "mondo salad," with iceberg lettuce, chickpeas, cucumbers, black olives, cherry tomatoes, sliced carrots, hard-boiled eggs, and bean sprouts, topped with Thousand Island dressing for my mother and Wishbone Italian for my sister and me.

My mother does not hurry in the kitchen. She is, shall we say, thorough. She cubes butter with a dinner knife a single pat at a time. The way she eyes and levels cups of flour, you would think she were transferring gold dust. Her drawn-out manner of doing things had sometimes been a tension point between us, but that October, her pace was perfect. Maybe because it allowed my own slowness to feel not so far off from the way of the world; maybe because her tremendous care was more important than any efficiency. My mom moved at my speed without comment—a kindness I hadn't always extended to her—and when she took twice as long as necessary to wrap my PICC line in plastic before my bath to keep moisture and infection out, I was grateful. When she smoothed and tucked and smoothed and tucked the bedsheets I'd be crawling right back into, I was glad.

She cooked for me, too, a strange task in those days since nothing tasted right. Any number of things were to blame: the brain injury from the initial hemorrhage, the aftereffects of the anesthesia, the infection, the antibiotics, my damaged sense of smell. The blandest cereal was sickeningly sweet, chocolate tasted like metal, and the mere sight of anything green—broccoli, spinach, even lettuce—made my skin crawl. My mother was on it, with batches of chicken soup and a palatably gray mushroom-beef-barley stew. I ate what I could, which wasn't much. Anyway, what I really wanted to do was cook.

One night, despite the fact that I could barely stand long enough to brush my teeth, I decided that I wanted—needed—to make dinner. I told my mom and she didn't hesitate. She picked up a pen, dug a scrap of paper from her purse, and transcribed the list of ingredients that I called out from the sofa. Mushrooms, cream, some frozen peas, though the thought turned my stomach. We had pasta and lemons already. When she got back from the market, she helped me into the kitchen. Eli was over by the sink, and he turned when I walked in. He looked happy to see me, but nervous, too, and very tired. It was great, he said, and weird, to see me back in there. The light felt bright, and I made it through three mushrooms, just washing, not even slicing them, before my legs grew heavy, my head light, and nausea flooded my chest. Eli helped me back to the sofa, and my mother finished preparing the meal. I think I might have slept. I wish I could say that those three mushrooms felt like a victory, but really what I felt was fear. *Three mushrooms.* I had to get back in there.

Lemony Pasta with Morel Mushrooms and Peas

The dish I set out to make that night was inspired by some pasta with morel mushrooms and fresh peas that I ate on my twenty-seventh birthday. Eli and I were living in San Francisco at the time while I was a visiting graduate student at UC Berkeley. With the birthday, the semester coming to an end, and our return home to Cambridge approaching, we were feeling celebratory and up for a splurge. We made a reservation at Chez Panisse, Alice Waters's restaurant on Shattuck Avenue.

Morels are difficult to describe because of how singularly delicious they are. They're woodsy and wild, you might say, arboreal in the way of hazelnuts and pine, succulent like meat. I'd never tasted one until that night, and I was thrilled by how much there was to taste. I did my best to re-create the pasta dish at home and it became part of our permanent rotation. It's best in the spring with morels and fresh peas, but we make it year-round with cremini or shitake mushrooms and frozen peas. If you use cremini or shitake mushrooms, you'll need to cook them for a few extra minutes to get them brown and crisp around the edges.

½ pound morel mushrooms (or cremini or shitake mushrooms; see above)

1 teaspoon Diamond Crystal kosher salt

½ pound (227 grams) dry linguine

2 tablespoons unsalted butter

Sea salt flakes, like Maldon, to taste

1 cup (150 grams) fresh or frozen peas

2 tablespoons fresh thyme, chopped

Zest from 1 lemon

¼ cup heavy cream

1 tablespoon extra-virgin olive oil

Freshly ground black pepper, to taste

Juice of ½ lemon, plus more to taste

Fill a large bowl with cool water and prepare the morels: Slice them in half lengthwise, swish them around in the water for a few seconds to loosen any grit—not too long; you want them to absorb as little water as possible—fish them out, pat them dry, and lay them out in a single layer on a dry towel. (If you're substituting cremini or shitake mushrooms, skip the bowl of water and wipe them clean with a damp paper towel instead. Then cut them into ¼-inch slices.)

Bring a large pot of water to a rolling boil and add the kosher salt. Add the linguine to the boiling water and give it a stir to keep the strands from sticking. Cook until just shy of al dente. (The pasta will finish cooking in a hot pan later on.) Drain the pasta and set aside.

Meanwhile, melt the butter over medium-high heat in a 12-inch pan. When the butter foams, add the morels, taking care not to crowd them in the pan. If your pan is small, you may need to work in two batches. Sauté the morels for six minutes, stirring occasionally.

Sprinkle with a pinch or two of sea salt flakes, and cook for another 1 to 2 minutes, until lightly brown, crisp around the edges, but still tender. Transfer them to a bowl and set aside.

Turn the heat down to medium, add the peas to the pan, and cook for 1 to 2 minutes (3 to 4 minutes if your peas are frozen), stirring once or twice. Return the mushrooms to the pan, stir in the thyme and lemon zest, and cook for 30 to 60 seconds. Add the boiled pasta and mix gently with the morels and peas, scraping up any brown bits from the bottom of the pan. Pour in the heavy cream, swirl it around the pan, and remove the pan from the heat. Add the olive oil, some sea salt flakes and freshly ground black pepper, to taste, and lemon juice, and mix gently. Taste, and add more lemon juice, if necessary. Serve immediately.

Makes enough for 3 to 4.

CHAPTER 21

Home Is a Verb

I was home but I wasn't. This was our apartment. Same red table, same bench, same sofas, same chairs. Same smell, presumably, though I wouldn't have known. The difference was me. I was sicker now, and my home only reminded me of that. The chair in my office demanded that I take a seat and turn on the computer, but I couldn't sit up for more than a few minutes at a time. I couldn't look at the bright screen without a lump of nausea lodging itself in my chest or read a page of text without my eyelids slamming shut. Everywhere I looked, I found evidence of my own absence, even as I stood right there. Loud things had gone silent and things that moved stood still: the mixer on the counter, the squeaky oven door, knives and napkins, notebooks and pens.

Before I'd gotten sick, I'd touched these objects every day. They were the tools I used for work and for play. From where I sat propped up on the sofa, a helmet on my head and a PICC line in my arm, they felt like artifacts of a previous life.

I didn't say a word to Amy about any of this when she arrived that first week in November after my mom went home. I didn't have to, because she knew.

Home is a verb. It's not only where we live, but how. I learned this as a little girl from Amy by watching her in her own home—especially in the kitchen.

Amy's kitchen and how she ran it were among the first things I noticed about her. The room was more like a studio of sorts, with its tools and towels and three kinds of flour. She kept her sugar in an old tinted glass canister with a metal lid and funneled whole black peppercorns into a ceramic mill. Her spoons were wooden, her pots heavy and worn. At eleven years old, I had never seen anything like it. I hoped that someday I'd have a kitchen like that, too.

Amy made uncomplicated meals that left you feeling the good kind of full. Her food, like everything about her, was straightforward, exactly what it seemed. A salad of black beans, red onions, cilantro, and corn cut straight from the cob. Grilled chicken with parsley and lime. Long before I'd ever heard of Chez Panisse or Alice Waters, I learned from Amy that the best food is food that tastes like itself, simple and clean. A potato at its utmost is a potato; a green bean, a green bean. To cook, Amy taught me, is only to help our ingredients down the path toward becoming their truest selves. It's no surprise then that she is a champion of vinaigrette, whose very function is to amplify what's already there. Splashed with vinaigrette, beets taste beet-ier, leeks, leek-ier.

Making vinaigrette is easy, but before Amy, I'd never seen anyone do it. She'd start with a near-empty Grey Poupon jar, spoon in some oil, then some vinegar, sort of measuring, sort of not. She'd screw on the lid and shake and taste, shake and taste, adjusting accordingly, usually in the direction of vinegar. Then she'd add some parsley or chives, a minced shallot, whatever she had on hand. I was thrilled by the efficiency of it: how those scrapes of mustard helped emulsify the oil and vinegar into a uniform dressing, how a jar at the end of its life had one more job to do.

Things happen fast in Amy's kitchen, though she never seems to hurry. She just moves quickly, casually along, from the cutting board to the stovetop, from the mixer to the oven door. Each task takes only as long as it takes. I hadn't known this was a way to be.

Amy taught me that butter should soften on the counter before it hits the table, how to toast pine nuts in the oven and say your own name out loud with proper exasperation when they burn. She was the first person I'd ever met who believed in cooking for its own sake. She'd page through a magazine, spot a cake, and bake it, for no other reason than that it was something she wanted to do.

I loved flipping through her recipe file, a binder thick with photocopies, torn-out magazine pages, and newspaper clippings that peek out on all sides. She stores it flat on a shelf in the cupboard above the oven, and when you pick it up, you have to squeeze so that its guts don't slide out onto the floor. You might think there is no method to it, but from constant use, a natural organization has developed based on what she likes to cook and what our family likes to eat. Recipes made most recently and most often gather at the top of the heap. Recipes made for a holiday meal, she slides back into the pile together, informal family histories of July Fourths and Thanksgivings.

Amy is the one who showed me that even when it seems like there's nothing good around to eat, there almost certainly is. Thaw a tub of chicken broth, open a can of tomatoes, empty the crisper drawer: soup. Fold last night's greens into omelets, chop a lone scallion into a nub of soft cheese. Grab a box of crackers, maybe a bunch of grapes. You have lunch.

Yes, home is a verb. To feel again that my home was mine, I'd need to set it back in motion. Amy understood that, so when she showed up in Cambridge that November, there were suddenly things to do. She made sure of it.

Rearranging furniture was at the top of the list. Amy is notorious for the pleasure she takes in moving things around. A bed turned ninety degrees and pushed back against the far wall, a dresser here instead of there: a new room. We decided to tackle the office-kitchen-overflow room (the one that drove me nuts). Amy and Eli nudged a filing cabinet into position, then lifted the long wooden sidebar away from the wall and slid it up against the windows. I shuffled around, taking stock, relieved by the movement, the newness, the extra floor space.

Amy spotted the philodendron in the other room. It had grown too big for its pot and was shrugging its leaves up and over onto the table. Amy suggested a several-block walk to the hardware store for soil and a larger pot, and I prepared myself the way I once had for my long Sunday runs. A few bites of food. Some sips of water. I tied on my running shoes, and Amy grabbed me a Gatorade from the fridge. We moved slowly, stopping twice so that I could rest and drink.

Back at home, I lay down on the sofa, the muscles in my thighs twitching from fatigue. Amy spread some newspapers on the floor right beside me. She crouched down, dug out the plant and its roots, transferred it to its new home, and pressed the soil into place. As she brushed off her hands, she looked up, and a puff of satisfaction blew through me.

Amy's Potato Salad

Until I met Amy, potato salad meant mushy peeled potatoes, maybe some celery and onions, and lots and lots of mayonnaise. Amy took a different approach, mixing skin-on red potatoes with crisp green beans and tossing them with scallions, chopped basil, and a mustardy vinaigrette. Over the years, I've tweaked things here and there: radishes instead of scallions; some combination of parsley, chervil, chives, and tarragon in place of basil. I've added hard-boiled eggs, too, which make me feel entirely justified in helping myself to a big bowl of this potato salad and calling it a meal. I like to eat it for dinner with the potatoes still warm—they're nice against the cold, snappy beans—but it's great from the fridge, too, for picnics and packed lunches.

You can boil your eggs for this recipe however you like to boil your eggs. My method is to put the eggs into a pot large enough so that they lie in a single layer, cover them with cold water by an inch, bring to a boil, then immediately remove the pot from the heat, cover with a tight-fitting lid, and let sit for 9 minutes. When the timer goes off, I fish out the eggs with a slotted spoon and drop them into an ice bath to stop the cooking. I recommend starting with eggs that are a week or two old. They're easier to peel than fresh ones.

For the vinaigrette:

    6 tablespoons olive oil

    3 tablespoons red wine vinegar

    2 teaspoons Dijon mustard

    ½ a large shallot, finely chopped

    1 tablespoon of chopped fresh herbs, any combination of
        parsley, chervil, chives, or tarragon

For the salad:

> 2 pounds red waxy potatoes, scrubbed under cold running
>   water and quartered
> 1 tablespoon red wine vinegar
> Diamond Crystal kosher salt
> 1 pound green beans, washed and trimmed
> 6 radishes, washed, dried, and thinly sliced
> 5 large eggs, hard-boiled and quartered
> Freshly ground black pepper

Combine all the vinaigrette ingredients in a jar with a tight-fitting lid, shake well, and set aside.

Put the quartered potatoes into a large pot and cover with cold water by an inch. Add a few generous pinches of kosher salt, bring to a boil, then reduce to a simmer. Cook, stirring occasionally, until the potatoes are fork tender, about 10 minutes. Drain the potatoes, transfer into a large bowl, and toss immediately with 4 tablespoons of the vinaigrette. Meanwhile, bring a second pot of water to a boil, salt it, and fill a large bowl with water and ice cubes. Blanch the green beans in the salted boiling water for 60 seconds, then transfer them to the ice bath.

Dry the beans and add them together with the sliced radishes and quartered hard-boiled eggs to the potatoes. Add the rest of the vinaigrette and mix gently. Serve right away, or chill it first if you prefer.

Serves 6.

CHAPTER 22

Doing the Math

On Amy's last evening in town, I wished out loud that I could bake an apple pie. The presidential election was the next day, and we had friends coming over to watch the television coverage. An apple pie seemed fitting.

Amy had only a couple of hours before leaving for the airport, but soon she was cutting cold butter into flour, flicking ice water at the shaggy heap, and patting it into disks. Eli peeled apples. Amy's cousin Sue Lena arrived to drive Amy to the airport and she picked up a peeler, too. My major contribution was holding myself upright in a chair wedged into the kitchen doorway and watching the pie take shape.

It was my grandmother Louise's pie, the apples seasoned simply and splashed with brandy and just enough lemon to help them hold their shape. My grandmother swore by Oronoque frozen piecrusts and kept a neat stack in the freezer in the garage. I'd updated the recipe with a homemade bottom crust and a crackly sugar shell-like lid in place of the one on top. From my chair in the doorway, I told

Eli how to make it: Melt the butter over a low flame. Stir in the sugar, then the flour and nutmeg. He tipped the pot in my direction so I could sign off, then painted the soft paste over the bare fruit. When the oven door snapped shut with the pie inside, it was time for Amy to leave.

"I don't want you to go," I said, wiping my eyes with my knuckles. When we hugged, my helmet clunked against her skull. She gave me four quick pats on the shoulder, her signature "there-there."

"I'll come back," she said. "We'll rearrange more furniture."

Soon after Amy left, the pie came out and Eli placed it on a rack to cool. I stared. Without its aroma, it didn't seem real. It was like seeing a picture in a glossy magazine or an image on TV. For a moment, I actually thought I could smell it, but no. My brain had been fooled by a lifetime of memories that knew just what the scent should be. This pie smelled like nothing.

It's hard to explain what it's like to smell nothing. We have the word "silence" to describe the opposite of noise, the complete absence of sound. But what's the opposite of scent? As far as I know, there isn't a word for it.

Smelling nothing is not the same thing as not smelling anything. I think that's why I'd known right away that something in my nose had gone wrong. You won't smell anything in an odorless room, but you will still detect something inside of your nose, something you'd never notice, let alone think to identify as an actual sensation, if you have never felt its absence. At least I never did. For a smelling person, air has weight, and while you can't smell weight, you can feel it. Much more so than the missing odors all around, the absence of this weight told me every day that my sense of smell had not returned.

I drew my face in close to the pie and inhaled. Still nothing.

But the hot steam on my cheeks worked my memory and there they were again, the outlines of scents: apples, cinnamon, brown sugar. I imagined my grandma Louise crouching by her open oven door, checking on her pie. I could conjure the scent of her, too. Like blueberries, first night's sheets, a screen door in the breeze.

She and my grandfather lived just outside of Hartford, Connecticut, up on a hill that had no grass, only trees. It was a long rectangle of a house, low-slung like a highway motel, a single floor that, because of the hill and the two-story drop from the wraparound deck to the ground, felt lodged high among the branches. The nineteenth-century writer and designer William Morris said, "Have nothing in your house that you do not know to be useful or believe to be beautiful." I think my grandparents must have lived by this rule. The décor was midcentury modern, lots of clean, straight lines, plenty of open space. My grandparents traveled to sixty-eight countries together over the course of their marriage, and the treasures they'd brought home were on display all over: a life-sized wooden rocking pig in the living room by the piano, a painting of a naked man smoking a long black pipe over the sofa, and, my favorite, a full miniature orchestra carved from polished stones under glass in the den.

When we'd visit, we'd come in through the garage, usually late at night. I'd squint into the fluorescent light and step into the kitchen. It was our landing pad. The Formica counters and metal cabinets were blue, the walls and floor were white, and the ceilings were the highest I'd ever seen in a house. On the island across from the sink there would always be a basket of fruit with a Post-it note stuck to one of the plums that said, "Washed." My grandmother would be standing next to it, and I'd run to her and press my forehead against her cheek while she'd hum-grunt into my ear, the same sound she'd make when eating sweet corn. "Hi, pussycat," she'd whisper. I'd breathe her in, and when she let me go, I'd inhale again and smell something else. It was the scent of arrival, the way our noses tell us, even in the absence of a scent we can name, that we've walked through a door and are now someplace new. Because even without a cake in the oven or flowers on the table, there's skin and dust, the faint aromatic echoes of everyone and everything that's passed through, a scent that's nondescript but for the precision with which you can remember it in your own nostrils.

My grandma was terrific in the kitchen. She made a killer zuc-chini bread, applesauce by the gallon, and jammy little cookies called coconut walnut delights all from scratch. She could cook. But she also knew how not to, and when not to so that she could get to the eating part sooner and with less fuss, and generally have more fun.

My grandmother was a big believer in the kitchen shortcut. That doesn't sound like the most flattering way to describe a woman who was serious about food, but it all depends on how you under-stand the word "shortcut." It's easy to think that shortcuts are for lazy people or people who can't do any better or are okay with second best, but that wasn't my grandmother at all. There's an art-istry to cutting corners, to knowing which ones are dispensable and which ones have to stay. Call it intuition or very good taste (I think the two are related), my grandmother had it. Her shortcuts were about being smart, efficient, and direct, exactly as she was in any case, and not only in her kitchen.

Shopping meant going in with a list of precisely what she was after. I never saw her browse. The summer before my junior year of high school, she marched me into a small clothing store and an-nounced, "We're looking for a pair of jeans with plenty of room in the rear." I fought back tears that night as I told Amy what had happened, but when I walked into school the following month wearing the best-fitting jeans I'd ever had, I felt like a million bucks.

This was why my grandmother loved to shop. It wasn't materialism that drove her, at least not in the shallow sense. It was the awareness that whether we like it or not, the physical objects that we surround ourselves with, the clothes on our bodies, the crackers in our pantries, the art on our walls, are an extension of who we are.

Some people might have a usual sandwich, something they order again and again so that, although all they've done is to consume what's on their plate, they become known for it. Grandma Louise was that way with a lot of things. She had a habit of finding something in a store or a restaurant or a grocery aisle and making it her own. The chocolate mint candies in the crystal jar by the piano, the sugar cubes with delicate flowers made of frosting painted on. She got her corn from a woman known as Mrs. Shmutz. *Shmutz* means "dirt" in Yiddish, and I'd say that my grandmother liked buying her corn from a woman whose hands bore evidence of the farm where it was picked, but honestly, I think what she really liked was how the Mrs. Shmutz moniker made that corn a "thing," something special and, by way of her profound appreciation of the kernels on those cobs, hers. Everything else was cow corn, she said.

All of this is to say that my grandmother took as much pride in the products she purchased as she did in what came out of her own oven. She knew that something didn't have to be homemade to help make a home.

So I don't think she would have minded that when I think of her kitchen, I remember mostly what she bought. Like the mini pecan rolls in white boxes, tied with string in the way that forms a plus sign across the lid. If the string was loose I could squeeze my hand into the box and slide one out, scraping my wrist against the box's edge. I knew that my grandmother didn't make those pecan rolls, but I thought of them as hers. They were more crust than crumb, burnished, caramel-candied knobs that fit in the palm of my hand. These rolls, my grandmother's rolls, were from William Greenberg's bakery on the Upper East Side. She had discovered them once on a trip to New York City, and since then she would bring them back several dozen at a time for herself and her friends, who were hooked on them, too. The pecan rolls, the mint candies, the whitefish salad she bought for Sunday brunch—the affection I felt for all these things taught me to never underestimate the power of a well-purchased edible.

Years later as a freshman in college, I'd think of her while shopping for student potluck meals. I'd stand in front of the refrigerated case, scanning the rows of hummus, baba ghanoush, and vegetarian chopped liver. The handles of my plastic basket would cut into my hand as I contemplated the relative merits of each tub. I had no kitchen, not a fork or a knife to my name, but when I pulled something of my own choosing off the shelf, a little piece of that dinner became mine.

My grandmother was nineteen years old when my father was born and forty-eight years old when I was. As a kid, those numbers thrilled me. I had the youngest grandmother of all my friends, and I was constantly doing the math. When I graduate from high school, she'll be sixty-six! When I graduate from college, she'll be seventy! I could have a kid before she's eighty. And because in our family people live on and on, she'll have another decade or two to go! I knew four of my great-grandparents, and three of them lived until I was in high school and college. That was normal, to me. But when I was twenty-three years old, and my grandmother was seventy-one, she died. It was all wrong. In my family, you're supposed to get more time. I thought Grandma Louise was the kind of person who lived until a hundred, as if that were a "kind of person" at all. I thought I was, too.

When I was visiting my grandfather a few years later, right after Eli and I were engaged, I found her wedding dress in the basement and put it on. It fit perfectly, as though it had been tailored precisely for my body—for my slender wrists and waist, for my bony shoulders and small breasts. There was plenty of room in the rear.

My doctor had said that my sense of smell would not recover, and I believed him. That was before I knew that doctors sometimes say things like that when actually, they don't really know. It's rare, but olfactory nerves do sometimes recover.

I suspected as much one day, sometime in November, when I walked into the lobby of our building with Eli and felt a rush of something curl up through my nose. I didn't smell it as much as I felt it swirling in my nostrils, pressing against my sinuses, and I had no idea what "it" was. I froze. I asked Eli if there was something in the air, if he smelled anything. "Yes," he said, "wet paint."

A few weeks later, Eli came home with sushi, and when he opened the bag, I said, "Oooh, smells cucumbery," as if it were the most natural thing in the world. I didn't even realize what I was saying until the words spilled out of my mouth. I was getting better. My sense of smell was coming back.

Louise's Apple Pie

I like to use two or three different kinds of apples in this pie, some tart and crisp, like Granny Smith, Honeycrisp, or Macoun, and one

or two of a juicier, sweeter variety, like McIntosh. That way the filling is pleasingly fluid, without oozing all over your plate. The crackly
sugar shell here is adapted from a recipe in Ruth Reichl's *Comfort
Me with Apples*.

Now, let's talk piecrust.

It's simple, in theory. Cut butter into flour and add just enough water to form a cohesive dough. That's how I did it for years, making sure
to follow the rules: cold butter cut into pea-sized chunks, large enough to
visibly marble the dough when flattened beneath a rolling pin. That
butter would melt in the oven, leaving air pockets between layers of flour
to form a nice, flaky crust. Mindful of gluten development—too much
means a tough crust—I'd add as little water as possible and take care not
to overwork the dough. It all made sense to me.

But cutting butter into flour is imprecise. Every time you do it,
there's variation in how much dry flour, completely loose from butter, remains in the mixture. That means variation, too, in how much
water you'll need for the dough to come together. Most piecrust
recipes list a range of water amounts because it depends. You learn
to adjust the water by a tablespoon here and there, and with a little
practice, your piecrusts turn out great.

What if you're new at this, though, and you'd like to get it right
on your very first try? For this book, I wanted a recipe with exact
measurements that would lead to a perfect flakey, buttery piecrust
every time. Even if you've never made a piecrust in your life.

I found exactly that in J. Kenji López-Alt's column "The Food
Lab" on the website Serious Eats. Kenji's secret lies in a "fat-flour
paste," as he calls it, which eliminates variation in the flour-butter
mixture. You make the paste by incorporating the butter into just two-
thirds of the flour, processing it in a food processor or cutting, rubbing, and squeezing it by hand until the mixture is the consistency

of Play-Doh. (You don't have to worry about too much gluten developing from overmixing at this stage. The proteins in flour need water to form gluten, and you haven't yet added any.) This fat-flour paste—essentially flour particles completely coated in fat—functions completely *as* fat. You then add the remaining bit of flour and a set amount of water that no longer varies batch to batch because you know exactly how much flour you're dealing with. It's brilliant and produces the best piecrusts I've ever made.

I always recommend measuring by weight instead of volume when baking. Here especially, since the volume measurements are a little fussy. Note that a scant ½ cup in this case means removing only about a teaspoon or so from the cup.

For the pie dough:

> ¾ cup plus 3 tablespoons (118 grams) + a scant ½ cup (59 grams) all-purpose flour, divided
>
> 1 tablespoon granulated sugar
>
> ½ teaspoon fine sea salt
>
> 10 tablespoons (142 grams) unsalted butter, cut into ¼-inch cubes
>
> 3 tablespoons cold water

For the filling:

> 2½ pounds (5 to 7 medium) apples (see headnote)
>
> ¼ packed cup (50 grams) dark brown sugar
>
> 1 tablespoon cornstarch
>
> 1 teaspoon cinnamon
>
> ¼ teaspoon fine sea salt
>
> 1 tablespoon fresh lemon juice
>
> 2 tablespoons apple brandy, like Calvados

For the topping:

½ cup (1 stick; 113 grams) unsalted butter, cut into pieces

¾ cup (150 grams) granulated sugar

¾ cup (94 grams) all-purpose flour

½ teaspoon nutmeg

Make the pie dough:

Stir together the ¾ cup plus 3 tablespoons (118 grams) flour, sugar, and salt in a medium-sized bowl. Add the cubed butter to the bowl. Use your hands to rub, squeeze, and squish the butter together with the dry ingredients to form a homogenous, not-at-all-sandy fat-flour paste with the consistency of Play-Doh. It will take a few minutes. Cover with plastic and chill in the freezer for 10 minutes.

Remove the fat-flour paste from the freezer and spread the dough around the bowl with a rubber spatula. Add the scant ½ cup (59 grams) flour and work it in with your hands until it's just incorporated. Sprinkle with the water, then fold and press the dough with the rubber spatula until it comes together into a ball. Form the dough into a 4-inch disk, wrap tightly in plastic, and refrigerate for at least 2 hours.

Alternatively, you can make the dough in a food processor. (It's faster, but you end up with more dishes to clean.) Combine the ¾ cup plus 3 tablespoons (118 grams) flour in the bowl of a food processor and pulse twice. Add the cubed butter, and pulse until the flour is fully incorporated and the dough begins to clump around the blades (25 to 30 pulses). Spread the dough around the bowl with a rubber spatula, sprinkle with the scant ½ cup (59 grams) flour, and give it 3 to 5 short pulses. Transfer the dough to a large bowl, sprinkle with the water, and continue with the by-hand directions above.

Prepare the filling:

Rub together the dark brown sugar, cornstarch, cinnamon, and salt in a large bowl. Wash, dry, but do not peel the apples, and cut them into ½-inch slices. Pile the apples into the bowl on top of the sugar mixture, sprinkle with the lemon juice and brandy, and mix gently with your hands.

Assemble the pie:

Preheat the oven to 425 degrees.

Remove the pie dough from the fridge, and let sit until rollable but still cold. Flour your counter, and roll out the dough with a rolling pin into an 11-inch circle. Transfer the dough to a 9-inch pie plate. Crimp or flute the edges, if you'd like. Pile the apple filling into the shell—you'll have a huge heaping mound, but it will shrink down in the oven—and put into the fridge while you make the topping.

Make the topping:

Melt the cut-up stick of unsalted butter in a small saucepan over medium-low heat. Add the sugar and stir well. Turn the heat down to low and add the nutmeg and flour, stirring to form a thick paste. Remove from the heat, grab the filled pie from the fridge and, using a rubber spatula, spread the paste over the apples. You don't want to cover the apples completely; they should peek out here and there. This "venting" keeps the apples from steaming and turning to mush.

Bake at 425 degrees for 15 minutes, then lower the temperature to 350 degrees and bake for another 35 to 40 minutes, until the pie is golden brown on top and bubbling. Let cool to room temperature, or just above, before slicing to give the filling a chance to set up.

Serves 8 or more.

CHAPTER 23

They Cooked

The day before I left the hospital in Burlington, I'd spoken with my friend Hila on the phone. "Jess, my darling," she said, in her thick Israeli accent, "when you get home, we will take care of you. Whether you like it or not, we will. This is what is going to happen."

Poor Hila had no idea what she was getting herself into. Nor did any of my other friends who, like Hila, were dead set on figuring out what I needed and how to give it to me. They took mornings off from work to escort me to doctors' appointments and held my hand during needle sticks and ultrasounds. Hila drove me to the hospital one morning with a big orange jug of my own urine, carried it inside, then took me out for lunch, cracking jokes the whole way. Sunny stopped by with books on tape. Caroline sent crystals. David and Amy came over on Halloween Eve with their three little girls, the five of them dressed as Iron Maiden, and rocked out in our living room on invisible guitars. Faraway friends wrote letters, sent mix CDs, and a subscription to Netflix. They told me their news.

Sarah was falling in love. Sarit was pregnant. With twins! Mary walked me around and around the block, then sat rubbing my shins and the back of my head where I still had all the feeling.

And, of course, they cooked.

Every night, someone and something would show up at our door. There were Lila's chocolate truffles and Elisha's cookies. Rachel made vegetable croquettes and Liba a pot of her curry. I didn't have a taste for much of it, but I was relieved to know that Eli had something to eat, and that it was good.

Then sometimes, my own hunger would surprise me. I'd be curled up on the love seat in my usual unhungry state, hear a knock at the door, and some food would appear that would wake my appetite right up. It happened first with bean soup. My friend Jonathan dropped it by one day, just something he'd thrown together, he said. It smelled wonderful. I spotted kidney beans and navy beans. They were perfectly cooked, with delicate skins stretched tightly around plump, tender middles. I took a bite. The soup tasted of meat despite not containing a scrap of it. The broth was thick and smooth like gravy, and the beans were creamy inside, like chicken liver mousse. I could feel my body rushing to accept it, my hunger spurred on by the consumption of food, and not the other way around.

Hummus from our neighbor David had the same effect. He once told me how he made it, soaking and cooking the chickpeas, then peeling every last one before blending them with sesame paste into the smoothest purée. He'd fill two wide, shallow bowls with the still-warm hummus, nestle hard-boiled eggs, olives, and pickles into the drifts, and carry them down the hall to us on a wooden tray. We'd scoop it into our mouths with oven-warmed pita from David's favorite Armenian bakery and, when the bread was gone, eat the rest of the hummus off spoons, like leftover frosting.

I was a guest in my own home those days, eating other people's food off plates that belonged to me. Once I was strong enough, I was a guest outside my home, too. Friday nights with our friends were back on.

We went to Eitan and Julia's, as before, but now we brought only ourselves. In this and many respects, I was a terrible guest. I'd spit food into napkins and push vegetables around on my plate. My taste buds were still up to no good. Yet Julia made feasts. A buttery mushroom soup flecked with thyme, salads with olives and feta, giant potato pancakes sliced like pizzas, bird after bird after bird. When she hit upon something I enjoyed, she'd pack up the rest to go.

One of these things was farro, a tender Italian grain that feels nice to bite into. I'd heard of it, but never tried it until that night at our friends' table. Julia had cooked up a pot and mixed it with peas, which tasted funny to me, but the farro itself was perfect: chewy, lightly sticky, with a flavor that was nutty and bright. No one blinked when I picked out the peas and ate only the grain. Nor did they mind when, wiped out from the act, I retreated to the sofa, uncapped my disfigured head, and flattened myself along the cushions for the remainder of the meal.

Being sick, it turns out, is an education in the art of guesting. I didn't see it that way at the time, likely because I didn't know that there were important things still to learn.

The phrase "gracious host" rolls off the tongue. We all know what it is to be one. What it means to guest with grace is trickier, because it's not what it might seem. A good guest, we think, is an easy guest. A considerate one. She arrives on time with a bottle of wine or maybe a gift, some chocolate or homemade jam. She asks what she can do. She wants to help. She insists.

What these best of intentions miss is the most basic thing of

all: that a good guest allows herself to be hosted. That means saying, "yes, please," when you're offered a cup of tea, instead of rushing to get it yourself. It means staying in your chair, enjoying good
company and your first glass of wine while your host ladles soup
into bowls. If your host wants to dress the salad herself and toss it
the way she knows how, let her, because a host is delighted to serve.
To allow her to take care of you is to allow your host her generosity.
I'd always been too distracted by my own desire to be useful to understand this. I got it now.

I missed hosting a lot. I missed the gathering of thoughts that
happens when you're deciding what's for dinner, the turning around
of the menu in your mind, rotating one thing in, one thing out,
simplifying, paring down. I missed making lists. I missed the order-
ing of time that hosting entails. I missed knowing with any degree of accuracy what I could accomplish in a set amount of minutes
or hours, being able to hurry up if I needed to, or stand at the
stovetop for a few minutes more if the mushrooms were slow to
brown.

Since moving to Cambridge, Eli and I had hosted a Chanukah
party every year. We invited everyone we knew. Eli would spend
days in the kitchen frying up potato latkes, the regular kind plus a
few batches of sweet potato curry, my favorite. We'd cut crudités
and make savory spreads, mashing herbs into goat cheese and yogurt, whipping feta with roasted red peppers. Eli would make cranberry applesauce, and for my part, I'd bake: carrot cake cupcakes
with cream cheese frosting, Mexican wedding cookies, and Marcella's butter almond cake, of course.

That Chanukah would be our fourth in Cambridge. "Join us,"
we wrote on the invitation, "for an evening of food, friends, and
fire, as we celebrate survival against all odds." The message would

have been appropriate on Chanukah any year; this year, we felt it all the more.

It was important to me to do it up right. We couldn't scale back. That would feel even more depressing than not doing it at all. (Fortunately, these were the years before we added homemade toffee to the list, and mini chocolate tarts, and molasses sandwich cookies.) We would need help, and Eitan and Julia were ready. They peeled potatoes over paper bags while Eli chopped onions in the kitchen. Meanwhile, I drew a party map as I had each year, pairing bowls with dips and platters with desserts, diagramming where on which tables each dish should go and which utensils we'd put out to serve them. The party map had always been our key for moving things swiftly along in the last hours before people arrived. This year, it was especially useful. I could plan out the entire party, and others could make it happen.

When it came time to bake, Eli joined me in the kitchen. I did what I could, scooping and measuring and missing the bowl, my one eye playing tricks on me as I went. When I got tired, I'd sit and read the recipe aloud, and Eli would take over the job. My frosting powers gravely diminished—again thanks to the nonseeing eye—I passed the job along to the others. Everyone was so careful, so generous in their efforts to do things exactly as I would have. Eitan turned out to be a natural, sweeping the spatula around the edges of the cupcakes to form tidy white caps and pressing a single walnut down into each one.

Smells had been returning slowly for weeks, in one nostril, at least. Eli had tested me with the contents of our spice rack after I'd smelled the cucumber that night. I'd closed my eyes and sniffed each jar. There was often something there. Something, though I couldn't tell just what it was. Or I could tell, I was sure, and I'd be totally wrong. "Bubble gum!" I'd insisted, over and over, until I opened my eyes and saw the jar of cinnamon in Eli's outstretched fist. It was a surprise and a relief, then, to smell the latkes as they fried, the applesauce simmering away, to smell the cinnamon smelling like cinnamon.

The party was familiar and fun. Then fatigue hit hard at the end of the night and I had to lie down. I was embarrassed slinking off to the bedroom, but a few friends followed and climbed up with me onto the bed. Sarah propped a pillow behind my back; Adena brought me a cookie and a cup of tea. We finished out the party right there, my friends hosting me again in my own home—on my own bed!—only I no longer thought of it that way. The English words "guest" and "host" live in opposing camps: the inviter and the invitee; the welcomer and the welcomed; the provider and the provided for. In other languages, there is no such divide. The French *hôte* means host *and* guest. Context assigns the meaning. That night, I was both.

Sweet Potato Curry Latkes

Sweet potatoes are lower in starch than the "regular" potatoes typically used to make latkes. That means a wetter batter. To get a crisp edge on these, you'll want to squeeze the excess liquid from the batter as you form the latkes, so that they're as dry as possible when they hit the hot oil. I get the best results frying latkes in a cast-iron pan, but a stainless steel pan will also do the trick.

For our Chanukah party each year, Eli makes ten times this recipe, and relies on my grandmother Louise's freezing and reheating technique, which turns latkes into a terrific make-ahead food: Instead of draining the finished latkes on a paper towel immediately after cooking, allow them to cool on a baking sheet lined with foil. Then freeze the latkes in gallon-sized Ziploc bags. They will keep in the freezer for up to one month. When you're ready to serve the latkes, heat them for 15 minutes in a 400-degree oven. The excess oil will spill out of the latkes onto the pan, and they will refry a little. *Then* you can place them on paper towels to drain any excess oil before serving. Your latkes will be as crisp as they were when they first came out of the pan.

This recipe is adapted from Joan Nathan's *Jewish Cooking in America.*

¼ cup (32 grams) all-purpose flour
¼ cup (32 grams) cornstarch
2 teaspoons granulated sugar
1 teaspoon brown sugar
1 teaspoon baking powder
¼ teaspoon cayenne pepper
2 teaspoons curry powder
1 teaspoon cumin
2 teaspoons fine sea salt
Freshly ground black pepper
2 large eggs, lightly beaten
1 pound sweet potatoes (about 2 potatoes)
Peanut oil, for frying (canola oil works too; if that's what you
    have on hand)
Sour cream and apple sauce for serving, if you'd like

In a large bowl, whisk together the flour, cornstarch, sugars, baking powder, cayenne pepper, curry powder, cumin, salt, and a few grinds of pepper. Add the lightly beaten eggs and stir to form a thick batter.

Fit a food processor with the grating disk. Peel the potatoes, and quarter each one lengthwise. Then cut each quarter in half lengthwise, so that you end up with 8 long, fingerlike pieces. This slender shape will produce the most even shreds. Vertically feed the sweet potato fingers through the grater, and stir the resulting shreds into the batter. If you don't have a food processor, use a box grater to coarsely grate the potatoes by hand.

Pour a ½-inch layer of peanut oil into a 10- or 12-inch pan—don't skimp!—and place over medium-high heat for about 3 minutes, until a test fleck of batter sizzles upon contact.

Use your hands to squeeze out the liquid from about ¼ cup of batter, form the batter into a ball, and drop into the hot oil. Repeat, spacing the latkes an inch or so apart. You don't want to crowd them. Flatten each latke a bit with a spatula, and cook for a couple of minutes on each side, until crisp and brown. Place the finished latkes on a paper-towel-lined baking sheet to cool and drain. (Unless you're freezing them to eat at a later date. See my note above.)

Taste, and season with additional salt and black pepper if necessary. We serve these with sour cream and homemade cranberry applesauce.

Makes about 15 latkes.

CHAPTER 24

Food Blog

I've never been very good at having nothing to do. I like deadlines and action items, making lists and crossing things off. Without a project, I get itchy. (Those closest to me might use a slightly different word.) Take the end of every graduate school semester. Relief sticks around for about a day after the final paper is complete, only to be replaced by the feeling that something is off, but I can't put my finger on what it is. Perhaps I'm coming down with something? Or there's something important I'm supposed to be doing? If only I could remember what. I typically go around like this for a few days, miserable, clueless as to *why* I'm miserable, until Eli—gently, carefully, wearily, I'm sure—spells it out precisely. "Babe," he says, "you need a project."

By the end of December, more than four months after the aneurysm had ruptured, that was truer than ever. I needed a project. Returning to my graduate work was the most obvious contender. My comprehensive exams had been postponed, but they'd come around eventually. I decided to try to study.

When I told my family about my plans to get back to it despite my medical leave, they said I should take things slowly. Maybe it's better to wait, they said, but I didn't want to. It was about more than having a project this time. The only way back to myself, I figured, was to pick up where I had left off as soon as I possibly could. So I reached for the book on imperial Russian history that I had been reading before the rupture, and opened to the chapter I had marked months earlier with a purple sticky tab.

I don't know what I expected. I guess I imagined myself getting swept up in the social policies of Tsar Nicholas I, relishing the stories of Jewish writers and the work they produced at the turn of the century. That's how it had always been for me when I would read this stuff. Now I felt locked out. I could read the words, but they wouldn't stick. I'd make it to the bottom of a paragraph, only to climb back up to the top and start again. Then I'd fall asleep. Was this the "lack of concentration" that my doctors had warned might hang around for the next six months? Had my brain been damaged after all? Was I physically still so far from good health that the work was truly too hard?

For the first time in my life, there was not a single thing that I was "supposed" to be doing. There were no paper deadlines or readings to finish for class. There were zero expectations. All I had to do was keep breathing, and people practically cheered. I'm sure there's something very Zen that one could say about this, about slowing down, stepping back, "just being." But doing things is important. Creating things matters. It's not that we live, but how, that makes us who we are.

"Why don't you start a food blog?"

My friend Megan has a way of tossing off questions like this with the utmost nonchalance, questions that turn out to be big ones.

"A what?"

"A food blog," she repeated.

This was January 2009. Food blogs had been a thing for half a decade, but I had no idea. I'd heard of blogs, of course, and vaguely knew what they were, but I don't think I'd ever even uttered the word "blog" out loud.

Megan is my best friend from college. She started off as Eli's, then, lucky for me, he shared. I actually didn't know her well at all when we were in school. Megan was Eli's friend, the beautiful one with the bright eyes and pixie cut who had danced professionally in New York before starting her freshman year. I'd met her a few times at Eli's place, but it wasn't until senior year that Megan and I took the same seminar on epic literature, were equally slayed by Derek Walcott's *Omeros*, and became friends ourselves.

Every week, Megan sat at the end of the long seminar table directly opposite our professor. She took notes with a mechanical pencil on plain white printer paper that she'd slip into a manila folder at the end of class. When she got especially worked up about a line in the text (which was often), she'd rake her fingers through her short hair and grab the top of her head so that her elbow pointed straight out into the room. Then she'd furrow her brow so deeply that her eyes would nearly cross and say something freaking brilliant.

I remember the first time I got the impression that we were maybe starting to be friends. We were on the bus, on our way with some classmates to our professor's house for an end-of-semester dinner, when she said something about my commenting style in class, about how the thoughts "bubbled out" of me. She said it in a manner so loving, even then, as though she got a kick out of me and just plain appreciated the way I was. *Oh! She likes me back!* I remember thinking. *This awesome person likes me back!*

Every year, Megan came to visit us wherever we were. To Seattle, where we brought her down to the market for grilled cheese by the water; to Cambridge, where she helped us eat our way through my first buttermilk-biscuit-baking bender; and San Francisco, where I supremed grapefruit after grapefruit for us to eat with avocado and bitter greens. She was there when I rounded the corner onto the West Side Highway in New York for the final stretch of my half marathon. She rode her bike alongside me, waving and cheering as I ran.

Now here she was again, with me and my helmet, sitting on the floor by the sofa, telling me to start a food blog. I'd been saying how I missed my studies, but couldn't seem to get back in, how in any case, I missed my everyday even more, especially in the kitchen. Sweeping the excess flour from the top of a measuring cup, unlooping a saucepan from the pot rack above my head, bringing a knife down with enough force to chop an onion in two. I missed waking up early, comfortable in my bed and in my body, contemplating the leftovers in my fridge and a second life for them beneath fried eggs; I missed braiding challah dough on Friday afternoons, carrying a heavy stack of dishes and a fistful of silverware to the table, standing around in the kitchen with Eli at the end of the night scraping plates, rinsing glasses, wiping down counters.

Megan had put it all together. It was important, she said, to spend those days doing something I loved. If I wanted to be in the kitchen, that's where I should be. If my everyday was what I needed to find, I should go and get it. A blog would be a place where I could gather the bits of normal life that were slowly sprouting up again and make something of them, a place where I could show up and do something. "And it would be fun," she said.

So I typed "food blog" into Google, blinked at the two million hits that popped up on my screen, and started clicking around.

Recipes, photographs, stories. One jewel box after another. The whole thing was a revelation: people sharing food and stories *on the Internet*, like one sprawling dinner party, tables and chairs for miles. The next day, I typed some words into an empty white text box, hit publish, and marched into the living room feeling as though I had just invented the Internet. Eli gave me a quizzical look.

"I started a blog," I said. I called it Sweet Amandine after my favorite almond cake and kicked things off with a post in celebration of toast, mostly because I could make it myself. It had just started tasting good again. I love toast. But a food blog needs more than toast to feed it. I would have to get cooking. That was the whole point, of course. I longed to be back in the kitchen. I also feared it.

I had felt something similar when I was sixteen, just learning to drive. Everyone I knew in high school couldn't wait to get their license. Not me. The thought of sitting behind the wheel of a three-thousand-pound vehicle racing along at thirty-five, fifty-five, sixty-five miles per hour was terrifying. I'd have nightmares of driving off the road and wake up incredulous that humans had ever deemed driving safe at all, that there were no rails or grooves in the road to keep people from skidding off, and *la la la*, everyone was just okay with this?

The kitchen seemed equally treacherous now. Fire! Knives! Hot oil! Blades and mixers that spin! I felt a rush of adrenaline every time I stood beneath the pot rack, wondering if my helmet would protect me should the whole apparatus come crashing down. To calm myself, I'd think of Eli hanging from the stud in the ceiling a few years earlier and remind myself to trust him, that the pot rack was secure.

This matter of trust was really at the heart of it—trust in myself, most of all. I didn't know how to. My newly broken eye kept throwing me off. I was never quite sure where my body ended and the rest of the world began. I'd lean in over the stovetop to lift the teakettle off the flame and clunk my helmet on the hood. My impaired depth perception had me catching only air when I'd grab for a knife in the block and dropping eggs from their shells onto the counter just to the left of the bowl. This was the kitchen where everything had once felt automatic. That I now had to think, slow down, take extra care made me feel clumsy and frail.

The kitchen became my arena for testing myself physically. I'd page through my cookbooks and stack of rumpled recipes in search of ones that felt safe. My favorite buttermilk biscuits, for example. I misjudged the depth of the bowl as I sank the whisk into the dry ingredients and sent some of the mixture flying. I scraped it back into the bowl. My wrists ached from rubbing cold butter into flour with my fingertips, but wait, hadn't they always? The familiar discomfort brought me back to myself.

I went along that way, gauging the strength of my body with each recipe, reorienting myself in space at every spill and burned fingertip, as my brain remapped itself and my depth perception improved. Meanwhile, I figured out how to compensate, holding the rim of the mixing bowl with one hand and tapping it with the other to determine the bowl's position before I poured. I curled my fingers as far away from the blade as possible as I chopped potatoes for Sunday breakfast. I left the skins on the apples for a *tarte aux pommes* and took my time slicing them into thin half-moons.

When the making and the eating were done, I'd sit down and write. Often, after a few minutes of staring at the screen, my eyes would begin to ache and my neck would tighten with nausea. I'd wish I could unscrew my head, so heavy and big, and just lay it down beside me for a while. Every few sentences or so, I would take a break.

Sometimes, I would move to the sofa and close my eyes, string together the words for the next line in my mind, then make my way back to my desk and write some more. It might sound painfully slow, this limping, bit-by-bit way of writing, but as phrases became sentences became paragraphs, I felt like I was flying.

The tendons in my shoulders and groin ached, maybe because of the medication, maybe because of so much time in bed, maybe because of any number of things that no one bothers to figure out when you've been so sick, when there was pain that could actually kill you and that pain has been resolved. I would wake up in the middle of the night too uncomfortable to sleep, feel my mind speeding off into the darkness, fear closing in, and I'd know what to do. I'd think about squash. About cornmeal cherry scones. I'd think about how to package up a head of cabbage or a can of sardines on the page, how to get it all down in words.

It seemed whenever I'd enter the kitchen, I'd discover a story, one that would nudge me over to something more real and more permanent about my life than illness. They were the kinds of anecdotes and reflections about food that I had been shooting off to my family and friends in letters for years, the stuff of dinner table conversations and postdinner phone calls with Amy about soups and salads and olive oil cakes gone wonderfully right and horribly wrong. Only now, it no longer felt like small talk.

The stories I remembered, the stories I made, let me know there was a life beyond the narrow world of recovery. At their heart were the protective powers of kneading, salting, sifting, and stirring, because you can't be dead and do these things. There are no available statistics on how many people die each year while baking an apple pie, and I'd like to believe that it's because you can't. When you're cooking, you're alive. You've got no choice. To fry an egg is to operate with the perfect faith that you will sit down and eat it. To season it with salt and pepper is a statement that you will do so with pleasure, according to your taste. When you're sick and broken and sad and afraid, it feels good to think of a time when you weren't. It feels good to remember a life when you were hungry, when things tasted good, and to try, in some small way, in one small room of your home, to reenact it.

I baked lemon bars, the curd bringing to mind my first encounter with lemon meringue pie, tall and regal like my grandmother Marion who made it. I remembered the way I'd expected my spoon to sweep through the frothy meringue and how it bounced off instead, how I lifted the meringue from my slice like a lid and went after the lemon curd alone. I stirred pots of polenta, baked coffee cake, cookies, and tarts. I wrote about home, good neighbors, and friends. Unpacking groceries into the pantry, setting a pot of water to boil and a colander in the sink, toasting a lacy scatter of sesame seeds—this was my life creeping back in. Writing about these everyday things was my way of registering them, really seeing them, and believing in them once again. My way of saying, "I'd like to talk about something else now." I didn't mention my illness on the blog at all.

Being sick is like walking around with a microscope strapped to your face at all times with your own body squished beneath the slide. You don't look away, at first because you can't—you're too sick—and then because you're afraid that if you do, you might miss a symptom or a sign and die. That cooking shifted my attention away from myself was a tremendous relief. In the kitchen, I got to care again about the small stuff that's not supposed to get to you, but does when you're normal and well. Now, when the biscuits burned, it was my privilege to care. The twinge of annoyance as I whisked them from the oven was proof I was getting better.

Buttermilk Biscuits

There's a little place in Boulder, Colorado, called Dot's Diner. I have never been there, but someone named Kimberly McClain once visited, and was so impressed by their buttermilk biscuits that she wrote to *Bon Appetit* magazine to see if their editors could snag the recipe. They did, and published it in the October 2000 issue. I was a junior in college then, and a recipe that required only a bowl, a spoon, and a baking sheet was right up my alley, since that was more or less all the kitchen equipment I owned. I've tried other biscuit recipes over the years, but I always come back to Dot's.

3 cups (375 grams) all-purpose flour

2 tablespoons granulated sugar

4 teaspoons baking powder

1 teaspoon baking soda

1 teaspoon fine sea salt

¾ cup (1½ sticks; 170 grams) cold unsalted butter, cut into
½-inch cubes

1 cup cold buttermilk

Heat the oven to 425 degrees and line a baking sheet with parchment paper.

In a large bowl, whisk together all the dry ingredients (everything but the butter and the buttermilk). Drop the cubes of butter into the bowl and rub them into the flour mixture with your fingertips until the texture resembles a coarse meal.

Make a well in the center of the mixture, and fill it with the buttermilk. Stir just enough to form a wet dough. Don't worry if you end up with a bit of flour at the bottom of the bowl. Better to leave it than to overmix. Drop a packed ¼ cup of dough per biscuit onto the prepared baking sheet, leaving a couple of inches between each biscuit. Bake for about 15 minutes, until golden brown on top.

Makes 12 biscuits.

CHAPTER 25

The All Clear

Around the time I started Sweet Amandine, I read *How to Cook a Wolf*, by M. F. K. Fisher. She wrote it in 1942, when war demanded rationing, and rationing demanded that economy become the home cook's highest value.

With the war in full swing, the wolf at the door was hunger, the literal hunger that people faced on a rationed existence, but also the hunger for peace, for simple pleasures, and the authority to determine the nature of one's own appetite and feed it accordingly.

Government agencies encouraged the public to think scientifically about how they might cobble together their recommended vitamins and nutrients each day. M. F. K. Fisher urged her readers to take a different approach, rooted in the belief that eating well and eating affordably are not mutually exclusive. The key, she believed, was approaching the stove with all the powers of one's mind and one's heart. When war rages, it is the only practical thing to do.

And so, *How to Cook a Wolf* is a book about cooking with

courage and faith. It's about granting oneself permission to feast, re-ally feast, on whatever scraps you have before you, despite the wolf nearby—in fact, because of him.

I found myself nodding as I read. From my own experiences with a wolf of a different kind, I knew that she was onto something. To trust in your own aliveness, in your own ability to sustain and be sustained—there are times when there is no greater act of defiance.

There is a line from the second chapter of the book that I kept coming back to: "It is all a question of weeding out what you yourself like best to do, so that you can live most agreeably in a world full of an increasing number of disagreeable surprises." That, I was learning, is what it's all about. My entire life, I had asked myself, "What would you do if you could do anything?" It was an attempt to step back from the path I was on, to locate paths not taken—not yet anyway—and figure out what I wanted most of all.

But "anything" means anything, and possibility is noisy. I would come up with five, ten, fifteen competing answers, struggle to choose just one, and do my best to go after it, full speed ahead. When I got sick, the question of whether I should do one thing or some other thing fell away.

Recovery is an incremental process: a first meal at the table, a first tying on of shoes, a first walk around the block. Next steps are small, obvious, prescribed for a while. Then, one bright day, there is a moment when you can decide. Suddenly, what's next is up to you. Your mind is quiet, your body is willing, and you know with stun-ning clarity what you want most of all to get back. "What would you do if you could do anything?" wasn't it at all. Instead, I should have been asking myself something else all along: "What would you do if you could do nothing?" That, for me, for a lot of us, I imagine, was the real question.

* * *

People were reading my blog. They were leaving comments, sending e-mails, asking questions about my recipes and sharing their own. We talked about soup and scones; crisp roasted chickpeas; sesame noodles made with oil, soy sauce, and rice vinegar, and no peanut butter, thank you very much. We did not talk about my brain. They didn't ask me about my blind eye, insist that I sit down, or place a hand on my shoulder and tear up. As far as these people knew, I was just fine.

And wasn't I? By early spring, when people would ask how I was doing, I'd tell them I felt great, and mean it. "All better" is probably a stretch when you have a dent in your face the size of a deck of cards, but after feeling so bad for so long, "really much, much better" felt like practically the same thing.

It was all relative. Every few weeks, I was certain I'd arrived. "I feel better!" I'd announce to Eli over breakfast, fully believing that I did. Then a few weeks later, I'd think back to that breakfast and how slowly I'd still moved when clearing my plate. I'd remember the weight in my bones I'd felt by the end of the day, and revise: "Now I feel better." Then a few weeks later: "No, now."

I started preparing for my exams in earnest, and this time, it felt okay. It wasn't too hard. The only difference, I told myself, was that I was reading these texts with a hockey helmet on my head. I developed certain habits at my desk those days beneath the shelves of books nailed to my office wall. I would drum the roof of my helmet, my fingernails clicking against the plastic as I read. Hook a finger over one of the rubber loops that held the chin strap in place.

My first follow-up angiogram happened in March. We drove up to Burlington so I could have the procedure back at Fletcher Allen and I was glad about that. Fletcher Allen was where I had almost died, where I'd had the riskiest, most invasive of my surgeries, experienced the severest pain of my life, and lost half my vision to boot. Yet my memories of the place were fond. Everything had seemed under control at Fletcher Allen. I'd felt so taken care of there, safe. *Ah, the good old days in the neuro-ICU! The complete bed rest lest I bleed to death from inside my brain!*

I understood the strangeness of it, but I couldn't shake the feeling. Returning to Fletcher Allen felt like traveling back to a time when all that had happened since I'd left—the infection, the craniotomy—hadn't happened at all. I baked Marcella's butter almond cake, sliced it into wedges, and packed it up into two boxes made of thick Italian paper that I'd been saving for something special. One was for Dr. Tranmer. The other was for Dr. Linnell, the neuroradiologist who had performed my first few angiograms and would do this one, too. When I asked a question, he had a habit of saying, "Now, that's actually very interesting," before starting in on his answer.

"You know," I said to Eli as we drove up the night before the procedure, "if this hadn't happened, we never would have met these lovely people."

"You're crazy," he said and drove on.

They put you in a place somewhere between sleep and consciousness before the angiogram begins. I hadn't quite climbed back into my right mind when Dr. Tranmer came by my recovery room to tell us what they'd seen: The clip was holding steady. The residual aneurysm was gone.

The first part we'd hoped for. Expected, even, with Dr. Tranmer's encouragement. That was the whole reason we were there, I thought, to make sure the clip hadn't budged. The second part I didn't understand. *The residual aneurysm was gone?*

"It resolved itself," Dr. Tranmer explained. "That happens sometimes."

It does?

Between the pressure in the vessel returning to normal after the placement of the clip, and the healing of the vessel wall beneath it, apparently so. My mind wobbled through the grogginess and nausea to try to grasp what he was saying. I knew it was good news, but his actual words were lost in the postprocedure fog.

On our drive home, Eli repeated what Dr. Tranmer had said: This was an all clear. Once my head was back in one piece, I could do whatever I pleased. Marathons, pregnancies, and the resulting babies expelled from my body in whichever manner I chose. The scheduled years of follow-up scans and monitoring were canceled. I wouldn't need them anymore. Without a family history of aneurysm or any conditions that would predispose me to forming more, I was done. The risk from angiogram was actually higher than the risk that I'd ever have another aneurysm again.

The possibility still existed, of course, but no more than for anyone else on the planet walking around with a brain in her head. In fact, you might say that my position was even better than the rest of the population, since I had at least been scanned and knew for sure that my brain was clean. It all felt so unexpected, so unlikely. I made Eli tell me again and again.

Some combination of jubilation and relief is no doubt the appropriate response in this scenario. I tried to feel it. When I called my parents to tell them the news, I pretended that I did, certain that any moment I actually would. But I couldn't. I didn't know how to believe it.

For seven months now, all signs had pointed to illness. When I brushed my teeth, a bashed-in head stared back at me from the mirror. It looked as though my brain had taken a deep sucking breath in, pulling my temple and half of my forehead inside. My left eye was missing part of its socket. It looked bulgy and off. Without the piece of skull to contour my skin, my eyebrow stretched into an unnatural arch a couple of inches above where it should have been. I looked perpetually intrigued. Or surprised. Or maybe sinister. Definitely not okay.

The cavity inside my skull was no longer sealed. A sensation of pressure in my head came and went. This was a post-op thing, I was told, something to do with tissues healing and the blood flow finding its way back around. No cause for concern. Still, I worried. Hadn't these doctors been wrong before? I'd been granted permission to think of myself as well again—but it wasn't the sort of thing that someone else could grant. I'd berate myself for letting fear take over. I felt crazy.

"It's not as if you live by the sea but constantly have anxiety about being trapped on a mountain," my cousin Katie reminded me, "or are anxious about polar bear attacks." She understood that trauma is a real thing and urged me to be kind to myself, and patient. Time, she said, would help quiet the voices in my head.

But what about the voices outside? With my doctors' permission, Eli had mounted my bike on a stationary trainer in our living room and I had started to ride. When I told friends and family, they'd frown. "Just be careful," they would say, "don't overdo it." My heart would pound. *Careful of what?* They knew about the all clear. Did they not believe it? And if they, my best people, did not, should I? I'd remind them of what Dr. Tranmer had said after my angiogram. "Just be careful," they'd repeat, so I'd smile and do my best to console and convince them some more. My real task was to convince myself.

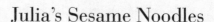

Julia's Sesame Noodles

I'd never been a fan of sesame noodles until I ate them at my friend Julia's table. The culprit? Peanut butter. It was a starring ingredient in the recipes I'd tried, and the sticky texture wasn't for me. Julia's noodles skip the peanut butter. They're slippery and light, mildly sweet. Her recipe was one of the first that I posted on my blog, and I still make it all the time. You can dress the noodles up, if you'd like, with chopped peanuts, sliced raw cabbage, grilled chicken, or tofu. My friend Stephanie adds julienned red bell peppers and carrots that she has lightly sautéed in sesame oil. The flavors of this dish don't fully come together until the noodles and sauce have cooled to room temperature, so you'll want to plan for that.

3 tablespoons sesame seeds
3 garlic cloves, minced
4 tablespoons rice vinegar
6 tablespoons soy sauce
2 tablespoons toasted sesame oil
2 tablespoons granulated sugar
1 pound dry angel-hair pasta or spaghetti
4 scallions, thinly sliced on the diagonal
Crushed red pepper

Toast the sesame seeds in a dry skillet on the stovetop, stirring frequently, for about 5 minutes, until the seeds are fragrant and take on a bit of color. Set aside.

Place the garlic, rice vinegar, soy sauce, sesame oil, and sugar into a small saucepan over medium heat and bring to a boil, stirring constantly. Remove from heat and set aside.

Fill a large pot with water and bring to a rolling boil. Add the pasta, and cook until al dente. Drain the pasta, transfer to a large bowl, immediately pour in the sauce, and toss. Let the noodles cool to room temperature. Gently mix in the toasted sesame seeds, the scallions, a pinch or two of crushed red pepper, and whatever else you'd like to add just before serving. Serve at room temperature or chilled.

Serves 4 to 6.

CHAPTER 26

More Than Enough

You can cook for one. A fried egg and toast, a potato with cottage cheese, a single artichoke, steamed. Baking, on the other hand? I don't care how big your sweet tooth is, you can't eat all those cookies alone. You bake to share.

Baking means you have more than enough: more flour, more butter, more eggs, to make more cake than you need for just you. It means you have something to give away. Baking is an act of generosity, and thereby an act of freedom, since to be generous is to be free from the smallness of thinking only of yourself.

Illness had made me dwell unnaturally on my own body and mind. I wanted to be generous again.

By the end of April, I was strong enough to stand and stir as long as I needed. I'd tackled quick breads, brownies, pastas, and salads. Now, with Eitan's birthday just around the corner, it was time for something more.

Birthday baking is so much fun. I love the precake song and dance, in which I get to ask precisely what you want, and you have to tell me. You hedge a little at first: "Oh no, don't bother. You don't have to bake for me." A beat of silence, then: "But if you *were* to," and we're off. Cakey? Fudgy? Fruity? Boozy? Whipped cream? Buttercream? Sugar glaze? Nuts? Taste is specific. It gives me rules to work within, and there's special pleasure in that: cobbling together the best parts of recipe A and recipe B to produce exactly what you desire.

Kasey wants layers. Jonathan wants pie. Hila wants citrus and a moist crumb, a "juicy cake," she calls it, with berries baked inside. My friend Sam wants Mexican wedding cookies, doughnut hole–looking things made from an eggless, butter-rich dough that's splashed with vanilla and specked with toasted ground pecans. You roll the cookies in powdered sugar while they're still warm, and they half explode, half melt in your mouth when you bite in. Eli's a birthday cookie man, too, oatmeal or chocolate chip, while Mary wants her cake to be *cake*, a dense, thick slab, she explains, a "cake you have to chew." She grabs at an imaginary cake of considerable weight floating in the air before us and squeezes to show how little it gives. A white cake, she says, or maybe something yellow, flavored with vanilla and slathered with jam? Hold the frosting, but whipped cream's okay, as long as it's not too sweet. For Julia, it's chocolate. "You know the kind of cake I mean," she says, and I do: dark chocolate, butter, heavy cream, eggs. You can keep your flour.

Now it was Eitan's turn. A couple of weeks before the date we'd scheduled to fete him, he and Julia came over for dinner. We were stuffed, flopped on the sofas, when conversation turned to cake. After the usual coaxing, Eitan's request was on the table: something strawberries and cream, preferably with custard, and a soft, white cake. That could mean only one thing, as far as I was concerned: cassata cake. *Cleveland* cassata cake, the kind I'd grown up on, made with custard instead of ricotta.

I was nervous. This was a layer cake. A celebration cake. And I was a sloppier cook than I'd ever been as I wrestled with my perception of where things were in space. I'd gotten a bit of sight back after the surgery to decompress my optic nerve, but not much. Mostly what I saw out of my left eye was blackness, with a narrow crescent of fuzzy vision in the periphery. I saw shapes and colors. I could even discern certain people and things. My ophthalmologist told me that the nerve had probably recovered as much as it could. It would certainly never be a reading eye, he said. I squinted at his chart with my right eye closed. I couldn't even see the big *E*.

Yet just as Dr. Tranmer had promised, while my sight did not improve, my vision did. My brain was remapping itself to understand the world with one eye. The brain is plastic, especially when you're young. People who are born with only one seeing eye or lose an eye in early childhood never notice a deficit at all in either field of vision or depth perception—because there isn't one. The brain figures out a monocular way to see it all.

At twenty-eight, I'd missed my chance for that kind of radical remapping, but I was still young enough (and lucky enough) that my brain did do a lot of the work for me. Except for when I was tired or rushing, I no longer sent mugs intended for the table crashing to the floor. The rest was up to me, to compensate for what I couldn't perceive with the way I operated.

I gathered the ingredients for Eitan's cake, read the steps, and felt the power of a recipe in a new way—how it takes you by the hand and tells you just what to do. A good recipe makes you brave. "One thing at a time," it says; step one, step two, and from this pile of ingredients, you'll make something delicious. Eitan's cake came together this way. First the custard, which I stashed in the fridge. Next, I baked the cakes.

How would I divide the batter evenly between the two pans? In the past, I'd simply poured. Now I used a ladle, doling out equal numbers of scoops. To check my work, I stuck a toothpick into the center of each pan, then lifted the toothpicks up and compared the batter lines. Good.

While the cakes baked and cooled, I sliced the berries and macerated them in sugar until they sat in a shallow bath of their own juice. It was time to split the cakes. As I sawed them in half with a serrated bread knife, I paid attention to the angle of my hand. I couldn't trust my vision to tell me if my cut was even, but I could feel the knife in my grip and know if I was holding it flat. I assembled the cake, three layers stuffed with custard and strawberries, then set out to frost it as best I could. I kept nearly gouging the cake with my spatula, or missing it entirely, stroking the air instead with whipped cream. My solution was to draw the handle of the spatula into my body and press it against my stomach, corresponding with the height of the cake. That spot on my body became my reference point for where the cake sat in space.

And soon it was done, a fluffy white cloud leaning a bit to one side, perhaps, little peaks and swirls of whipped cream that I hadn't managed to smooth beneath a crown of strawberries. Eitan gasped when he saw it, and as I cut into the cake and pulled out a wedge striped with custard and fruit, he giggled like a kid. Jonathan and Hila were there, too, and Eli. I eased slices onto plates and passed them all around. It was perfect. Flour and butter and eggs that could have become anything, transformed. We scraped our plates clean.

Cleveland Cassata Cake
(Strawberry Custard Layer Cake)

When I first started hunting around for a cassata cake recipe, I found one after another that called for ricotta cheese between the cake and strawberry layers. I was baffled. It was custard in the cake that I remembered from my childhood.

With a little more digging, I found that, while most cassata cakes are indeed made with ricotta, Corbo's Bakery in Cleveland has long produced a custard and strawberry cassata cake. Their Sicilian family recipe traces back a hundred years, and no less than chef Mario Batali has called it "the best cassata I have tried in the USA." Other bakeries and supermarkets in the Cleveland area took their cue from Corbo's and made their cassatas with custard, too.

This cake is a bit of a project in that it involves several components and takes some advance planning. To keep things manageable, I usually make the custard and the cake a day in advance and store them in the fridge. (Chilled cake is easier to split into layers, anyway.) I then macerate the berries, whip the cream, slice the cake into layers, and assemble the next morning.

Keep in mind before you begin that you'll want to chill the assembled cake for 8 hours before serving.

I used to make this recipe as a four-layer cake, but frankly it was all too much. It was hard to slice without making a mess, and the servings were impossibly large. I now assemble it as a three-layer cake and save the leftover layer in the fridge or freezer. It's nice to have around for a last-minute dessert of strawberry shortcake. Just whip some cream, slice some berries, and cut the cake into rounds with a biscuit cutter. It's great in an impromptu trifle, too. You will also end up with a little extra custard, but I assume you have a spoon and will know just what to do.

For the custard:

>   6 large egg yolks
>   ½ cup (100 grams) granulated sugar
>   2 cups half-and-half
>   ½ teaspoon pure vanilla extract
>   3 tablespoons cornstarch

For the cake layers:

>   8 large egg whites at room temperature
>   ½ teaspoon cream of tartar
>   ¼ cup (50 grams) plus 1¼ cups (250 grams) granulated sugar, divided
>   2¼ cups (271 grams) cake flour
>   1 tablespoon baking powder
>   1 teaspoon salt
>   5 large egg yolks at room temperature
>   ½ cup cold water
>   ½ cup vegetable oil
>   ¼ cup lemon juice
>   1 teaspoon lemon zest
>   1 teaspoon pure vanilla extract

For the strawberries:

>   2 pounds strawberries, divided
>   2 tablespoons granulated sugar

For the whipped cream:

> 2 cups chilled heavy cream
> 1 tablespoon granulated sugar

Make the custard:

Whisk together all the custard ingredients in a saucepan. Bring the mixture to a boil over medium-low heat, whisking constantly. Turn down the heat so that the mixture just simmers, and whisk until thick, 1 to 2 minutes. Transfer the custard to a bowl, cover with plastic, and chill for at least 3 hours, or overnight.

Bake the cakes:

Heat the oven to 325 degrees. Spray the bottoms (not the sides) of two 9-inch round cake pans with cooking spray, line the bottoms with cut-out circles of parchment, and spray the paper.

In the bowl of a stand mixer, beat the egg whites with the cream of tartar until soft peaks form. Add the ¼ cup sugar, and beat on high until the peaks are stiff but not dry. Set aside.

Sift the flour, the remaining 1¼ cups sugar, the baking powder, and the salt into a medium bowl.

In a separate large bowl, use an electric hand mixer on high speed to beat together the yolks, lemon juice, water, oil, zest, and vanilla until smooth. Fold in the flour mixture with a rubber spatula until just combined.

Using a rubber spatula and a very light touch, fold about a quarter of the fluffy egg whites into the egg yolk mixture. Then fold in the remaining whites. The goal here is to incorporate the egg whites without significantly deflating them. As soon as the egg whites are no longer visible, stop folding. (A streak or two of egg white is preferable to overmixing.)

Scrape the batter into the two prepared pans and spread evenly. Bake for 30 to 35 minutes, until the tops spring back when lightly pressed and a toothpick inserted into the centers comes out clean.

Leave the cakes to cool in their pans on a rack for at least an hour. When completely cool, run a knife around the sides to release the cakes, cover each pan with a wax-paper-lined plate, and flip. Lift the pans off of the cakes, and carefully peel back the pieces of parchment. Wrap the two cakes in plastic, and refrigerate at least 3 hours, or overnight.

Prepare the strawberries:

Thinly slice 1 pound of the strawberries lengthwise, ⅛-inch thick, and place in a medium-sized bowl. Sprinkle with the 2 tablespoons sugar, and stir. Leave the strawberries to macerate for at least 1 hour. Give them a stir once in a while. They will release their juices. Strain the berries, reserving the syrup. (Don't worry if you don't end up with much syrup. Some strawberries are juicier than others.) Meanwhile, slice the remaining 1 pound of strawberries lengthwise, ¼-inch thick, and set aside. These unmacerated berries are for the top of the cake.

Split the cakes, whip the cream, and assemble:

Remove the custard and cakes from the fridge. Using a long, serrated bread knife, carefully saw each cake into two equal layers. You'll only need three layers for this cake. Store the fourth, well wrapped, in the freezer for another day. Place each of the three remaining layers on a wax-paper-lined baking sheet or plate.

Whip the cream and sugar together until stiff.

Tear four 2- to 3-inch strips of wax paper and arrange them in a square on your cake stand or serving plate. Place one cake layer in the center of the square, with the four strips of wax paper partially sticking out on all sides. (The strips are to keep the plate clean from frosting. You'll remove them before serving, taking any smears with you.) Brush the top of the cake with half of the reserved strawberry syrup. Cover with 1 cup of the custard, then half of the sliced macerated strawberries. Top with the next layer of cake, and repeat: syrup, 1 cup of the custard, strawberries, cake.

Using an offset spatula, cover the entire cake with whipped cream. Arrange the sliced unmacerated berries in concentric circles on the top of the cake, and press them into the sides of the cake around the bottom.

Chill the cake for at least 8 hours, then bring to cool room temperature before serving.

Serves 12.

CHAPTER 27

Time-In

At the beginning of the summer, my surgeon told me he wanted to fix up my skull two whole months earlier than planned.

"Will August work for you?" he asked. I laughed out loud, wondering what on my calendar could possibly take priority over getting my head back in one piece.

He hadn't said that the early surgery date was the result of my doing particularly well, but when people asked, that was what I said. "Yes, it was supposed to be in October, but I'm doing so well that my surgeon wants to do it in August instead." It just felt so good to say it, to feel as though this time things weren't only going according to plan, but better.

The date was set: August third. We dubbed it "Humpty Dumpty Day," with surgeons in place of king's horses and men and my head the talking egg. My parents bought plane tickets. I told my department at school that I'd be ready to teach in the fall and knocked out two exams. I went in for 3-D scans so that the prosthetic piece could be fitted to my head. The end was in sight.

* * *

In June, six weeks before the surgery, Eli and I boarded a plane for Seattle. I took the window seat and leaned my helmeted head against the wall, plastic on plastic. It was actually nice, the way the thickness of the helmet kept my head propped at a gentler angle, easier on the neck. Eli was sleeping with one hand on his thigh when the tip of Mount Rainier poked up through the clouds. I put my palm on the back of his hand and slid my fingers between his.

When we touched down we went straight for provisions—Red Vines, cherries, Beecher's cheese, Copper River salmon, chicken, and lamb—then sped east into the Cascades. We were on our way to Lake Wenatchee, a couple of hours outside of Seattle, to a house that belongs to our friends Rich and Martha. They live with their daughters in the city most of the time, but spend long weekends and vacations at the lake, hiking, climbing, and skiing in the nearby mountains. That summer they would be traveling and asked if we might like to stay at the house while they were away.

We'd been out there once before, a few months after we were married when I went skiing for the first time. Eli had dressed me up in one of his orange ski jackets, a fluorescent green fleece turtleneck, and an extra pair of goggles, and signed me up for a beginners' class. I did okay. During the brief intervals I remained upright, anyway. The view from the chair lift was lovely, a nice distraction from the impending crash dismount that I managed to execute every time. It was perfect, Eli and I had joked: He'd nearly passed out after the required three-lap swim test in college, but I loved the water. If we ever had kids, between the two of us, they'd be covered for all seasons. I was a pro at après-ski, at least: hot chocolate at the lodge, then back to Rich and Martha's for apple pie.

Their house was classic Pacific Northwest, made of wood, slate, and stone. The rooms flowed one into the next, with windows that stretched up from the chattered wood floors all the way to the ceiling, framing the lake mere feet away and the mountains all around. It was an easy house to be in, minimal in a way that felt luxurious: neutral palate, exposed beams, spare furnishings.

The natural aesthetic had added power for me on this trip. As I'd grown stronger, I'd been taking off my helmet around our Cambridge apartment occasionally. Never in the kitchen, and never at my desk beneath the overstuffed bookshelves, but when the only thing above my head was ceiling—on the sofa reading with Eli, at the dinner table—I'd unbuckle the strap and give myself a break. Outside, it never left my head.

At Rich and Martha's, even inside felt like the outdoors. I'd stretch out along the window seat, take off my helmet, and feel free. A deck wrapped around the entire back of the house, and with nothing but a meteorite to come crashing down on me, I went bareheaded out there, too. It was my first time outdoors without a hockey helmet on my head in more than eight months.

This home was an open space, a safe space where I could be broken. And with Humpty Dumpty Day just around the corner, where I could begin to think about what it would mean to be whole again.

Down the road from the house was a trailhead at the base of a mountain called Dirty Face. We'd wake up early every morning and hike a little ways up and back.

I kicked at the uneven terrain to help me navigate the roots and rocks along the path. More than once, I stepped down into a ditch that my eye had missed. My teeth would clack together as my boot hit the ground. But I felt strong. I loved the way Eli's bare neck bobbed along in front of me, how he smelled faintly of sweat and sleep. I loved the monarch butterflies, the brush against my legs, the ponderosa pines and bigleaf maples overhead, the wild roses, mariposa lilies, tiny waterfalls, and narrow streams. Each day we'd go a bit higher, then return to the house for the day.

I liked looking in the mirror at the end of those hikes before I showered. I noticed things I hadn't seen since I'd been sick. My skin, smooth and clear, my cheeks flushed from exertion. My hair, though matted from the helmet, looked thick and full. It was strange and new how little I noticed the massive deformity alongside the other things I saw. I kept hearing what my surgeon had said, that with the prosthetic piece in place, I'd look good as new. At Rich and Martha's, I believed it.

This was a working vacation for us both. I'd photocopied articles and packed up my sticky tabs, highlighters, and a suitcase full of books to prepare for the remaining doctoral exams I planned to take before the surgery. Eli had brought his laptop and, after some climbing at nearby Icicle Creek, would check in with his office each day. We'd hike, study, work; he'd climb; and in the six or seven o'clock hour, Eli would light the grill. He was in charge of the protein and opening a bottle of wine, and I would handle the rest of the meal: bread, salad, and dessert.

Cooking there was fun. The one pop of color in the house of grays and wood tones was a deep red Viking oven. You had to wedge a tipped chair under the handle to get the oven door to shut all the way. Otherwise, it was ready for business.

On my first night there, I found Rich's bread recipe tucked between two cookbooks and got to it. The bread began as a wet dough that developed overnight and into the next afternoon with a long, slow rise. When I dumped the dough onto the counter, it clung to the bowl in strands and strings that I swept free with an oiled spatula. I cranked the oven as high as it would go. Then, after a final rise, I transferred the dough to a cast-iron pot, clapped on the lid, and baked it until the bread was swollen and brown. I was careful but no longer afraid as I shook it from the pot. It crackled as it cooled. Meanwhile, Eli finished the salmon on the grill. I tossed spicy greens with vinaigrette, sawed into the bread, and the crust shattered. We dragged slices through olive oil and salt and pressed squares of cheese into the soft crumb.

Each night after dinner, I would return to my perch on the window seat to read or write. Eli would build a fire, and we'd fall into bed a little earlier than we typically would at home. Then we'd wake up the next morning and do it all again.

At first, I studied all day long. The books on my exam lists were ones I'd selected myself and I was interested in what they had to say. Everything was as it should be—or getting close. I was doing it: studying, researching, preparing to teach. I was en route to my former life, just as I had hoped. But the pantry was stocked and the oven called, and where I really wanted to be was in the kitchen. I wanted to be making things, and while the biscuits baked and the pie dough chilled, to get some of it down in words.

Suddenly, the months I'd spent doing just that felt painfully temporary. Here I was, a few weeks out from my final surgery, the one that would close the door on the illness and injury of the past year. I was almost done at last—and wanting a little bit not to be. It was the strangest thing, this tug of longing for the days that I was still squarely in. The very days that I'd been counting down. There in that house on the water, something was happening. Something so quiet that it was barely perceptible to me. It was more of a stir than a shift, a breeze that swirls through a pile of leaves, holds them in the air for a moment, then sets them back down, the same pile, rearranged.

The evidence had been mounting. Pastas and tarts and tomatoes heavy with juice, tables full of friends, and writing about it all. This had been no time-out. All those months away from my studies and the life I had known: this had been a time-in.

So I gave myself over to it in that house by the water, cooking and writing with an urgency I hadn't felt before. "You're so happy," Eli said one night as he cleared the plates. "I think you should pay attention to that."

He was right. During those long months, food had called something up in me that needed calling, demanded things of me that my academic work had not. It had inspired me to make something of the everyday life around me, of my home and of my heart, to make something of myself. My kitchen wasn't the route back to the person I had been. It was the route to who I would become. Life didn't freeze when I flew off the treadmill that morning and neither did I. There was no going back, and for the first time I realized that I didn't want to.

A week into our stay, Megan arrived for a visit. We decided to hike Dirty Face all the way to the top, nine miles round-trip with a four-thousand-foot climb. We started early.

I felt strong, but uneasy. I told myself it was okay if I had to turn back. But as we hiked higher and higher, past the markers of every other morning's hike—the stream you had to jump across, the waterfall, the fallen tree that Eli called "our bench"—I knew we were going all the way.

The early trail snakes up along the mountain in tight, tree-lined switchbacks, then opens onto a long-abandoned logging road, wildflowers everywhere in bloom. It then narrows again into a dense forest path that carries you up along the eastern spine. The chin strap of my helmet was soaked with sweat by the time the trees began to thin.

As the trail disappeared into the flat, broken scrabble rocks of the final ascent, the view unfurled: blue water tossing off sparkling coins of sunlight, rolling green hills, mountain peaks etched into the sky. The bigness was sudden. Eli, Megan, and I wordlessly spread out from one another, each of us scrambling and crunching our way to the summit on our own. We stood for a moment and just looked. Lake Wenatchee and its tributary rivers stretched out before us. The Chiwawa Valley and the snow-capped Cascade Mountains. There was Glacier Peak, where Eli and I had gone backpacking years earlier, where he'd told me about the ring and I'd ducked into my sleeping bag, too happy to say a word. Eli grabbed me, picked me up, and swung me around. All three of us were laughing, teary, calm.

Then down, down, down we marched, back to the house. Eli and Megan jumped into the lake. I wasn't allowed to, presurgery, so I went for a shower, found the dough I'd left to proof in the fridge, and shaped it into disks for pizza on the grill. We'd picked up a giant sack of cherries at a roadside stand and I tore into it now, whisked together a batter of milk and eggs, and baked clafoutis. It was my first clafoutis, a category-defying dish that's a cross between custard, a pancake, and flan. The eggy batter puffed up, then sank back down, and the cherries slumped in their own private craters. We ate outside in bare feet, our plates on our laps, my helmet on the table beside me. "Is it crazy to look at me?" I asked Megan. I waited for her to verify that indeed it was, or worse, but instead she smiled and said, "I just see a happy Jess." The Pacific Northwest sky was bright well into the nine o'clock hour, and I felt whole in my brokenness for the first time.

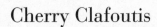

Cherry Clafoutis

The base for clafoutis typically involves only flour, milk, and eggs, but getting it just right can be tricky. You need enough eggs for the custard to set up, but use too many and the flavor is overly eggy and the texture turns gummy as it cools. To solve this problem, I've cut back on the eggs and added baking powder for a bit of lift. The custard comes together best in a blender, but if all you've got is a bowl and a whisk, use them, and get it as smooth as you can.

For the kirsch in this recipe, I like Trimbach. It's pricey, but since I only ever use a teaspoon or so at a time, a single bottle lasts a while. Kirsch works its magic on all manner of stone fruits and berries, by the way. Toss it with peaches before baking them into a pie or with plums destined for crumble to enhance the fruits' flavor. If you prefer, you can swap in amaretto or ½ teaspoon almond extract for the kirsch in this recipe. Clafoutis traditionalists get their hint of almond flavor by leaving the cherries unpitted. I tried that once, but worried so much about my guests' teeth that I've been pitting my cherries ever since.

1 tablespoon softened unsalted butter for greasing the pan
Granulated sugar for dusting the pan
2 cups (400 grams) fresh cherries, pitted
1 cup whole milk
3 tablespoons (38 grams) brown sugar
1 teaspoon baking powder
2 large eggs
1 teaspoon pure vanilla extract
1 tablespoon kirsch
¼ teaspoon fine sea salt

⅓ cup (42 grams) all-purpose flour
Confectioners' sugar, for finishing

Preheat the oven to 375 degrees.

Grease a 9-inch baking dish, cake pan, or pie plate with the 1 tablespoon butter. (Use the entire tablespoon so that the coating is thick.) Dust the sides and bottom of the dish with granulated sugar and shake out any excess.

Put the cherries into the baking dish and shake into a single layer. Combine the milk, brown sugar, baking powder, eggs, vanilla extract, kirsch, salt, and flour in the jar of a blender, and blend on high speed for 1 minute. Pour the batter over the cherries, and bake for 30 to 35 minutes, until the clafoutis puffs up and turns golden brown, and a tester inserted into the center comes out clean.

Serve at room temperature or chilled, dusted with confectioners' sugar.

Serves 6.

CHAPTER 28

Humpty Dumpty Day

There was a package waiting for me when we got back home from Seattle. A Humpty Dumpty doll carved from wood. His clothing was painted on, a red jacket with blue lapels. His legs, hinged at the knees and also red, dangled down from his egg-shaped body. My father had sent him in honor of the surgery that was now just three weeks away. I perched him on my desk as I studied for my last exams. Sometimes I'd absently stroke his head. It felt smooth, solid, strong.

The technical term for the kind of surgery I was having is "cranioplasty." The word made me think of papier-mâché. How in preschool, we would drag strips of newsprint through a flour and water paste and drape them around inflated balloons that we'd pop once the paste had dried. We'd draw faces on the paper "heads" that remained and stick on yarn for hair.

Cranioplasty has likely been around since ancient times, when surgeons used precious metals and gourds to repair injured skulls. The sixteenth-century physician Fallopius (after whom the fallopian tube is named) described the use of gold plate, and there is a record from 1668 that mentions canine bone. By the twentieth century, surgeons were using human bone from elsewhere in the patient's body to make repairs, and today, a prosthesis made of synthetic material is common. My prosthesis was custom made from a polymer based on the 3-D scans of my skull. The prosthesis was porous, so my own bone from the surrounding skull would grow right into it over time.

The plan, as I understood it: Have the cranioplasty on August third. Stay in the hospital for about a week. Recover at home for a month or so. Hang up my helmet, and get on with my life, looking and feeling as good as new.

The shape and location of the missing piece of my head would make the operation tricky. The hole was part forehead, part temple, part eye socket, part top of my skull. Because of the delicate facial curves and eyebrow positioning to consider, my neurosurgeon recommended that we consult with a craniofacial plastic surgeon and that the two of them perform the operation together.

It all seemed quite simple. The plastic surgeon examined me—that he seemed unimpressed by my deformity was a source of relief—and he agreed to do the surgery. The only thing we'd have to do, he told us, was to shift the date of the operation a few days up, or push it a few days back, to fit with his OR schedule. That afternoon, I spoke with the neurosurgeon's secretary, who said she would look into making the change. She sent me an e-mail a few days later: "All good to go for 8/3." The plastic surgeon would be able to make that date after all, she said.

My family arrived the weekend before the surgery. I wanted to feed them, so on Friday afternoon I walked the neighborhood alone to gather provisions, a few canvas bags looped over my shoulder, helmet on my head. At Hi-Rise Bread Company I picked up a flute, their version of a *pain a l'ancienne* made with a blend of white and whole wheat flours. Its crust is crisper than a traditional baguette; its flavor full. From there I walked along Huron Avenue, down the hill to Formaggio Kitchen. The cheesemongers sliced samples from plastic-wrapped rounds and offered them, still on the knife, for me to taste. Without precise enough depth perception to peel them from the blade, I stretched out my hand as casually as I could and let the mongers flip the portions onto my palm. Something creamy, something hard, something in between. Three chubby wedges wrapped in paper and sealed. I chose a bottle of white wine from the shelf beside the cheese counter. Olives. Slippery anchovies lifted from a bath of vinegar and oil. Then back up the hill and down another, through the square to the farmers' market, for peaches, cucumbers, and tomatoes at their height, swollen, seamy pouches of flesh, seeds, and juice.

I made Eli's aunt Leslie's gazpacho for dinner that night with its hallmark tarragon and cumin, flavors I'd never think to pair but which did each other right. With the spoils of the afternoon laid out on our red table, people served themselves, then sat wherever, anchovies, olives, cheese, and bread piled into their now-empty gazpacho bowls. Amy, my dad, and my brother, Caleb, were there, and my aunt and uncle, and Eli, of course. The next day, my mom and grandfather would arrive, and the day after that Eli's parents. Then it would be Monday, Humpty Dumpty Day.

Sunday evening I made a quiet salad of couscous and tiny green lentils that glistened like caviar as I rinsed them in the sink. I folded in what was left of some arugula from the fridge and the rest of the tomatoes, applied olive oil, lemon, salt, and pepper, and put out the bowl with a stack of plates for anyone who came by. Beside the salad, I placed a wooden board with thick slabs of banana bread lopped in half to make them easy to eat with your hands. I'd baked two loaves from the blackening bananas on the counter, one for Sunday and one for my family to have the next day while the surgeons put me back in one piece.

In my kitchen, banana bread is a food of departure. Before a few days or weeks away, I tend to view the perishable contents of my refrigerator and pantry as an edible checklist. It feels good, clever, baking bananas into bread, blending berries into smoothies, chopping greens into omelets, making delicious what would otherwise go to waste. Cooking is, on the one hand, an act of resistance to the coming departure. (I should be packing.) But as I empty out my fridge and sop up the last of what my kitchen has to offer, it is also an acknowledgment that soon, I'll be out the door.

Cooking before leaving home for someplace new means clinging to what's familiar before nothing is. It also means getting to eat something good, which is wise before a trip, in any case. There was no way of knowing how long I'd be away this time. *The doctors said one week,* I reminded myself, as I scored Xs into the bottoms of a few overripe peaches, lowered them into a pot of boiling water, plunged them in ice water, and slipped off their skins. But I was afraid it would be much longer. I quartered the peeled peaches, slid them into a Ziploc bag, and stashed them in the freezer. "I'll be back," the gesture said, "and I'll be hungry."

Whole Wheat Banana Bread

I adapted this banana bread from the Classic Banana Bundt Cake that appears in Dorie Greenspan's book *Baking: From My Home to Yours.* I halved the recipe to make just enough batter to fit a loaf pan, and swapped in some whole wheat flour to deepen the flavor. Instead of creaming the butter with an electric mixer, I melt it and fold everything together by hand for an especially tender, muffinlike crumb.

Ideally, the bananas for this recipe should be ripe past the point where you'd want to eat them straight from the peel. You're looking for plenty of dark brown spots—if your bananas are almost entirely black, even better—and some squishiness when you hold them in your hand.

Store the bread at room temperature, covered tightly with plastic. It will keep for a few days this way, and only improves with time.

Dry ingredients:

1 cup (125 grams) all-purpose flour

½ cup (57 grams) whole wheat flour

1 cup (200 grams) granulated sugar

1 teaspoon baking soda

¼ teaspoon granulated salt

3 ounces (85 grams) semisweet chocolate, chopped into small, irregular pieces (The largest chunks should be about ¼ inch.)

Wet ingredients:

1 large egg

1 stick (113 grams) unsalted butter, melted and cooled slightly

1 teaspoon pure vanilla extract

1 cup (235 grams) mashed overripe bananas (You'll need 2–3 medium bananas.)

½ cup (123 grams) plain, whole-milk yogurt

Preheat the oven to 350 degrees, and butter and flour an 8½-by-4½-inch (6-cup) loaf pan.

Whisk together the dry ingredients in a medium-sized bowl. In a large bowl, lightly beat the egg, then add the rest of the wet ingredients and stir well. Dump the dry ingredients into the wet ingredients, and gently fold with a rubber spatula until the flour mixture is just incorporated. Do not overmix.

Pour the batter into the prepared pan, and bake for 50 to 60 minutes, until a tester inserted into the center of the loaf comes out clean. Cool in the pan for 10 to 15 minutes, then carefully turn out the bread onto a rack. Cool completely before slicing.

CHAPTER 29

Luxury Head

Harvard Square was quiet in the 5:00 a.m. hour. The sky was still half sleeping, greenish pink around the edges. Eli and I could hear our shoes against the bricks as we walked. We went down into the T and caught the first Red Line train of the day. It was only three stops to the hospital, but by the time the train climbed aboveground with a view of the Charles River, the sky had ripened into daylight proper. I felt as though I'd been awake for hours.

"Ready, lady?" Eli asked.

This would be my third surgery. Fourth, if you count the decompression of the optic nerve on the heels of the aneurysm clipping. All of those surgeries had been emergencies, urgent, slice-and-saw responses to trauma, injury, and infection. This one was different. Except for the hole in my skull, I was fine. Totally healthy. *Wait, why was I having this surgery, again?* I mean, the helmet was annoying and all, but a mere inconvenience, wasn't it, compared with being cut open?

My mom and dad were already in the waiting room when we got there. I checked in, changed into a couple of johnnies, one with the opening in the back, the other in the front. I knew the drill. Cold snaps against my skin. Hospital bracelet.

I hopped up on a gurney behind a curtain and took off my helmet. Someone had left a thick folder of papers on the table, my medical records, and I flipped through them feeling like a snoop. I jumped when my family pushed back the curtain. "Hi!" I said, too loudly, and slapped the folder shut.

A nurse came by and said it was time to go. I asked to use the bathroom first, gathered up my gowns, and snapped my helmet back on. "Okay, so, um, be right back," I said brightly. I started toward the hallway, but my dad touched my arm and pulled me in close. "It's okay," he whispered in my ear, "this is a big deal."

"I know," I said, my voice catching.

"I know," he said back.

Eli came with me to right outside the OR, and the neurosurgeon met us there. "Now, there *is* a possibility that we won't be able to place the prosthesis today."

"What?"

Apparently there could be trouble pulling apart the tissues. Without my skull to keep them separate, my forehead and the outermost dura surrounding my brain had likely fused. If separating them took too long, they'd have to go back in with the prosthesis another time.

"When you see me in recovery, will you tell me right away if my head is back?"

"Sure," the doctor said. "But it's likely you won't be with it enough to remember." I was told before each surgery that I wouldn't remember the recovery room, but I always did.

"Please, just tell me right away," I said. "Will I see the plastic surgeon before we begin?"

"No, he won't be here until later. His job comes in at the end."

I awoke in the recovery room with the neurosurgeon standing over me.

"You did fine."

"Do I have my head back?"

"What's that?"

"My head. Is it back?"

He smiled. "Yes. Yes, it's back."

"Thank you. Thank you so much."

I was moved to a room and Eli came in as soon as they let him.

"Jess, your head is back," he said, first thing, in case I hadn't yet heard. I reached out and squeezed his arms and cupped my hands around his face. I just wanted to touch him.

"I know." I laughed. "The doctor told me. How do I look?"

"Like a person with a head," Eli said. "Looks great, lady."

We did it, I thought. *It's over.* I asked for a mirror so that I could see myself before the swelling set in. Yep, I was a person with a head. I swept my eyes over the face staring back at me. My forehead was in place, my eyebrows level. Something was off, though. My left temple. A golf-ball-sized dent was still there. I reached up to touch it and traced my finger along the now-complete eye socket. The edge of the bone felt unnaturally sharp where it dropped off into my hollow temple.

"Eli," I said, "my temple. Does it look not quite filled in to you?" He tipped my chin up with his fingers and stared at me, his mouth a straight line.

"Maybe. It's hard to tell right now. Could be that the surrounding area is already beginning to swell, and that's why it looks that way."

"Right," I said. "Is the plastic surgeon still here? I haven't seen him. I want to thank him."

Eli looked suddenly tired. "He didn't show up."

It took me a second before I could speak. "What do you mean?"

No one could say exactly what had happened or where the communication had broken down. A month later, at a follow-up visit, I would ask the secretary about it, and she'd say that she had made a mistake. That was all.

The neurosurgeon pointed out that it was impossible to know what, if anything, might have been different if the plastic surgeon had been there. Temporal wasting is common following craniotomies. Detached from the bone for so many months, the temporalis muscle atrophies. My doctor was right, of course. In an alternate universe where both surgeons were present, maybe something goes terribly wrong and I never make it off the table. But maybe, with the plastic surgeon there, I wake up all the way intact.

My mother stayed with us again for the first week of my recovery. I hung around the house for a few days, mostly because that was what I thought I was supposed to do. The truth was, I felt great. Which is to say, like a healthy person recovering from surgery. I'd never been that before.

I'd been home for four days when my mother and I decided to walk over to the farmers' market on campus. My first real helmet-free outing. I tied a navy blue bandana over my scar and pulled it awkwardly down over the remaining dent in my temple. I felt naked and self-conscious without my helmet, vulnerable, though my brain was better protected now than it had been in almost a year.

We cut through the park on our way to the market, and when we passed a game of ultimate Frisbee, my body switched into high alert. I instinctively moved to the far side of the path to give myself an extra second or two to react should an errant Frisbee glide uncomfortably close. I'd forgotten that I now had a skull to protect me.

We wandered among the stalls piled with tomatoes and zucchini, tiny raspberries, corn. We filled our bags. My mother bought a thyme plant for my kitchen window, a scoop of cherry lambic sorbet for me, and coffee ice cream for herself. We sat down on the steps of a building in Harvard Yard. I'd accepted a teaching fellowship for the semester and would walk into the classroom in three weeks. There was a lot to do before then.

"I want to bake something," I said.

I hadn't dared to say it out loud, but before leaving for the hospital, I had secretly challenged myself to bake challah my first week home. After my first surgeries, it had taken me months to regain the strength to produce the two braided loaves. If I could be well enough to bake challah this time after only one week, it would be proof that I was well on my way.

I started baking bread when I was in middle school. A friend of my mother's gave me a bread machine, and I used it to make terrible whole wheat bricks from bagged flour mixes. The thing that the manual called the baking pan was actually more of a bucket, a vertically oriented rectangle with a dough hook that snapped into place on the bottom. What came out were not so much loaves but towers that you would have to pry from the "pan," tearing a hole in the bottom where the dough hook had baked into the bread after the kneading cycle. We ate it warm with butter, and at least butter is nice.

After Eli and I were married, I tried bread baking again, this time doing everything by hand. I baked challah every Friday for Shabbat dinners, and before long I had it down. My hands worked and shaped the dough as if on automatic.

I adjusted my bandana as my mom and I stood up to go, and smoothed the hair on the top of my head. It was warm from the sun. *I have a luxury head*, I thought. At home I had everything I needed: flour, salt, yeast, oil, honey, eggs. That dent was just a battle wound. It was time to get on with it.

Five-Fold Challah

For years, the challah I baked was fine. Not great, though I was convinced it was. That's because we always ate it super fresh, still warm from the oven, when all breads, even so-so ones, taste like something special. Once cooled, and certainly by the next day, the bread would be just okay. Its flavor would flatten out and the texture would go a bit crumbly and stiff.

This challah is different, thanks to a tip from my friend Andrew Janjigian, a baker and editor at *Cook's Illustrated* magazine. Instead of kneading the dough, he said, try folding it. Then stash it in the fridge for a long, slow rise. With this technique, the gluten develops beautifully. The crumb is elastic and light, and the loaf pulls apart in fluffy wisps like cotton candy. The flavor is deep, almost buttery, though it's made with olive oil. And it's just as good on day two.

While this recipe takes a day or so from start to finish, it needs your attention for only a minute here and there over the first couple of hours. Then you leave the dough alone until you're ready to shape and bake it. I start the dough before dinner a night in advance, then go about my business at home, popping into the kitchen whenever it's time to fold.

I've included weight measures for the liquid ingredients here, because I've found it to be the simplest way to measure them for this particular recipe. With sticky, clingy things like honey and oil, it's fastest when you can measure directly into the bowl.

Please note that this recipe calls for instant dry yeast, not active dry yeast. Andrew explained to me the difference: Active dry yeast is coated with a layer of dead yeast that must be dissolved in order for the yeast to activate. That's why you have to proof it. Instant dry yeast, on the other hand, is all viable yeast. It's easier to use because there's no need to dissolve it in liquid. You just add it to your dry ingredients, and you're off. It's all I ever keep around. I buy the big red, white, and blue sacks of SAF-Instant yeast, which you can find online and in some grocery stores. Fleischmann's makes two instant yeasts, BreadMachine Yeast and Rapid-Rise Yeast, that are widely available in stores.

Dry ingredients:

4 cups (500 grams) bread flour
1½ teaspoons instant dry yeast
2 teaspoons fine sea salt

Wet ingredients:

2 large eggs plus 1 large egg yolk (save the extra white in a
    covered glass in the fridge for glazing later on)
¾ cup (190 grams) water
⅓ cup (75 grams) olive oil
¼ cup (85 grams) honey

For sprinkling, before baking (optional):

Flaxseeds
Rolled oats
Sunflower seeds
Pumpkin seeds

Whisk together the dry ingredients in a large bowl, and the wet ingredients in a smaller bowl. Dump the wet ingredients into the dry ingredients and stir with a rubber spatula until a wet, sticky dough forms. Cover the bowl with plastic and let sit for 10 minutes.

Peel back the plastic. Grab an edge of the dough, lift it up, and fold it over itself to the center. Turn the bowl a bit and repeat around the entire lump of dough, grabbing an edge and folding it into the center, eight turns, grabs, and folds in all. Then flip the dough so that the folds and seams are on the bottom. Cover tightly again with the plastic, and let sit for 30 minutes.

Repeat the all-around folding, flipping, covering, and resting for 30 minutes four more times. (I keep track by drawing hash marks in permanent marker right on the plastic.) The dough flops more than it folds in the first round or two. Then, as the gluten develops, you'll get proper folds. By the final fold, the dough will be wonderfully elastic, and you'll be able to see and feel the small pockets of air within. Pull the plastic tight again over the bowl and refrigerate for 16 to 24 hours.

Cover a baking sheet with parchment paper and set aside. Transfer the dough to a lightly floured surface and divide into six equal pieces. Roll into six strands, about a foot long and ¾ inch in diameter, dusting sparingly with flour when necessary to prevent sticking. (You'll want to add as little extra flour as possible.) Form two three-strand braids, and transfer the loaves to the prepared pan. Cover with plastic and let proof at room temperature for 2 to 3 hours, until the dough is noticeably swollen and puffed and bounces back very slowly, if at all, when you poke it lightly with your finger.

Preheat the oven to 375 degrees.

Remove the plastic from the loaves and brush with the reserved egg white. If you'd like, sprinkle with seeds. Poppy and sesame seeds are traditional challah toppings. I typically cover one with a combination of flaxseeds and rolled oats, and the other with sunflower seeds and pumpkin seeds, though lately I've been opting for no seeds at all.

Bake for about 20 to 25 minutes, until the bread is golden and gorgeous and a tester inserted into the center comes out clean. You can also check for doneness with a thermometer. The internal temperature of the loaves will be 190 degrees when fully baked.

Transfer to racks and let cool.

Makes 2 loaves.

CHAPTER 30

Don't Look

I was grateful when the semester began. It had been a strange four weeks since the surgery. I hadn't known what to do with myself, so it felt good to be back in an environment that prescribed my next steps for me: Pass out syllabi. Grade papers. Meet with students. I started my dissertation. I attended lectures and organized seminars. Sometimes, I'd mindlessly go to hang my finger on the strap of the helmet I was no longer wearing, and my hand would thump to the desk below. *This is me, getting on with it,* I'd tell myself. *This is what I am supposed to be doing.*

Every morning I'd inspect my head and my face, looking for improvement. *Is my scar a bit flatter? Has the swelling gone down? How is the bruising?* One by one, the signs of surgery disappeared. The dent in my head did not. It was an odd effect. I didn't look sick anymore. Just deformed. This was my face now.

Don't look. It doesn't matter. I turned away from the mirror when I brushed my teeth. *Don't look.* But sometimes I did. I'd glide my fingers gently down into my scooped-out temple and tickle the soft skin. If I pressed at all, it hurt. The spot was tender like a bruise. I looked at the top of my head. After the initial surgery to clip the aneurysm, my scar had been barely visible, a thin, straight line tucked neatly beneath my hair. But now my head had been opened twice more along that same seam, my scalp stretched repeatedly back into place and stitched closed. I had a landing strip, a half-inch band of permanent baldness across the top of my head. These things were not going away.

That there was nothing left to be done was supposed to be a good thing. Now the sense of finality had been turned upside down. There was nothing left to be done, all right. They'd fixed what could be fixed. I shouldn't complain, I told myself. The dent was in the squishy part of my temple and didn't pose a threat to my brain. The protective part of my skull was fully intact. My helmet sat in our bedroom closet on a shelf so high I couldn't reach it without a ladder. But the surgery hadn't felt like the end point I'd expected.

I went over and over the conversations with doctors and secretaries in my mind, trying to figure out what I could have done—what I should have done—to make sure the plastic surgeon was there. I had tried to be vigilant, smart, careful, polite, thorough, responsible, good. How could something have gone wrong *again*?

My doctors and friends liked to tell me how, even with the remaining dent, it was *soooo* much better than before. But really? Was that the bar? Was a skull that looked as though it had been attacked by a killer melon baller really all we had hoped to surpass?

I wanted to punch myself in the face for thinking these things. If I were more grateful, less shallow, stronger, wiser, if I had my priorities straight, if I had learned anything at all about what really matters from the previous year, if I were a better person, this stupid little defect would mean nothing to me. Maybe then I could look in the mirror and see my face, and not a reminder of my own near-death, my own brokenness, screaming back at me. I was healthy and helmet free. I was given the green light to run again. To have children. I was back in school. My brain was clean, the aneurysm gone. What was wrong with me, getting all worked up about a dent the size of a golf ball?

I called my dad. He said my feelings weren't about the remaining defect, not really, and he was right. They were about the whole long slog of it coming to an end, about having no more next steps, no upcoming tests or surgeries to keep me looking ahead and looking forward to becoming well again, bit by bit. There were no more bits. This was me, all patched up. I felt as though I'd been on a bus for thousands of miles, then dropped, alone, at the end of a dusty highway. I hadn't arrived anywhere at all, but there was nowhere left to go. *What had happened to me? What the* hell *had happened to me?* "You had to feel it sometime, Jess," my dad said. I didn't understand what he meant. Hadn't I been feeling it all along? Wasn't this the part where I was supposed to *not* have to feel it anymore?

Stop it. Just stop it. Stop crying. You're fine. I would will myself out of this: I had a weird-looking face. So what? I'd never been beauty oriented, anyway. All my life, I'd assumed it had to be one or the other. You were pretty or you were smart. You cared about looks or the important stuff.

Eli didn't believe me when I said the dent was no big deal. Even I didn't believe me. But, each in our own way, we pretended that we did. We wanted so badly for it to be true that everything was okay. If we could just stand back, keep quiet, and let time do its thing, shrinking and squeezing all that had happened into a mere blip in the larger context of a long and healthy life. If we could just hold tight.

Health. Family. Work. These were the things that mattered. I lunged for them. I shoved my nose into the yellowed pages of nineteenth-century books and newspapers. I wrote a paper. I translated texts. I did yoga and lifted weights. I started running again, too, though I feared it. Eli came with me, at first. We started slowly, running, then walking, then running again, as much as I could take. Soon, we were counting the miles. Each bridge along the Charles was a finish line: JFK, Western Avenue, River Street, BU. Sometimes panic would claw itself out of the box where I kept it and swipe at my heels. I'd notice an itch on my scalp and scan the trail to see who might come to my rescue if I collapsed. *The couple on the bench. The man with the dog. That girl on the grass has her cell phone out. She could make the call.*

I was starting to think again about becoming a mother, allowing myself to want it all the way now that the surgery was over. But was that right of me? Moms were supposed to be strong. Fearless. Moms are the Protectors, and here I was, unsure of whether I could even protect myself. Though my doctors insisted otherwise, I felt prone to breakage. I feared having a child and being too sick to care for her. I feared dying and leaving her without a mom.

Then other times, I felt strong.

One unseasonably warm evening in late October, I ran alone for the first time all the way to the Mass. Ave. bridge, over three miles from my front door. The river widens there, and when the autumn sun is low, the city of Boston glows orange and the water is liquid light.

"I think I'm starting to be ready," I told Eli when I got home. "Are you?" I was sure I already knew the answer. We'd had this conversation before, two summers earlier, one night in bed right before I got sick. His answer had been yes, and had stayed yes, as far as I knew. Trying to conceive was something we had looked forward to once we had learned it would be safe. My body just had to get strong enough again. I was the one we were waiting on.

Eli looked away and did what I call his "uncomfortable yawn," an unconscious move of his that buys him some time when he's about to say something hard. It starts out as a fake yawn with his chin jutted out to one side, then blossoms into a real one. I felt my chest tighten.

"We need to talk about your head," he said.

"No." I knew where he was going.

"I think we should go see the plastic surgeon. See if he can fix it."

"No way."

"Jess—"

"Are you crazy? Another surgery? No. It's just a stupid dent. I don't even care. I want to be a mom. I want to do this. I'm ready to do this."

"You do care." His voice was soft. "And you should."

"It's just my head. It's just my face." I was crying. "I can't believe after everything . . . The risks of another surgery . . . We know what can happen. I need you to understand."

"I don't understand."

I wanted to shake him. *We've escaped! We've made it! I can't go back.*

"Don't you at least want to know?" he pressed. "Find out if something can be done? I'm just talking about getting some information."

"Stop," I said. "Please stop."

We didn't exactly decide to "start trying." What we did was more along the lines of "stop preventing." Anything else would have felt too medical, and I needed this to feel like the opposite of medical. We'd had sex—careful, attentive sex—when I was still missing a part of my skull. Now we could lose ourselves again. Or, almost. I wondered sometimes when Eli closed his eyes if it was because he didn't want to see. Wherever his hands were, I felt where they deliberately were not: along the side of my face, my temple, my brow. Sometimes, when Eli would pull me close in the darkness, he'd accidentally brush his lips against my sunken skin. I'd shrink back from the soreness, then try to mask my recoil as a coy pivot, sliding my body into a different position alongside his.

I'd read somewhere that even under perfect conditions, when both of the relevant parties are as fertile as can be and timing is spot-on, there's still only a 33 percent chance of conception with each cycle. So it wasn't the not being pregnant that troubled me those first few months. It was the conversation we'd inevitably circle back to. If I wasn't pregnant, surgery was an option again. We would be eating breakfast, doing the crossword puzzle in bed, or driving up to a friend's wedding in Montreal, and Eli would get that look and yawn that yawn.

"Just think about it," he'd say.

"I have," I'd insist. "And no."

I was fine. Fine! Doing the work. Running the miles. Attending classes and giving talks. But back in the library stacks, in seminars about the very writers who had inspired me to go to graduate school in the first place, something wasn't right. I felt like I was moving around in a life that was two sizes too big and two sizes too small at the same time. At night a jolt of adrenaline would sometimes shock me awake, and I'd start sobbing, afraid. *But of what?*

All those months, the helmet had concealed the part of my head that was broken. Cruising the frozen foods aisle, sipping tea at a café with a hockey helmet on my head, I didn't look particularly damaged. I think I mostly just looked like a weirdo. "Hey, killer!" someone had called out as I stuffed my bag into the overhead compartment on our way to Seattle. Sometimes, I'd be walking down the street and hear a voice shout, "Safety first!" That my actual illness was invisible made me feel invisible. Now, with the helmet gone and a head that looked more or less like a head, I waited to reappear. Instead, I felt more invisible than ever. If the helmet had hidden my secret, my newly reconstructed skull, however flawed, hid it even better. *But I am still broken!* I screamed inside. I wanted no one to know. I wanted everyone to know. I said nothing.

Simplest Tomato Soup

I go through phases with recipes, making the same granola, for example, week after week, eating it daily. Then one morning, for no good reason, I stop. I eat eggs for breakfast, or Grape-Nuts, or toast. I develop some kind of amnesia that keeps me from knowing that granola ever existed. Until, months later, when I remember that it does, and off I go again on a mad granola streak, wondering how I ever got along without it.

This kind of ebb and flow in the kitchen creates a sense of seasonality beyond peaches in the summertime and apples in the fall. I remember who I was the last time granola came around, what I was doing, the book I was reading, the friend who came to town. And vice versa: When I think of that book or that friend, granola springs to mind.

When I was newly patched up but feeling broken still that fall, I made a lot of soup. One big batch on the weekends to stretch for as many lunches and dinners as I could manage. This simple tomato soup figured heavily in the rotation then. It's smooth, bold, and improves with age. I ate it all the time, after long hours in the library and runs along the river. I was also into a certain soda bread, a squat little loaf with a craggy crust; a nutty, faintly sweet flavor; and a compact crumb that slices well. It makes terrific toast.

1 large yellow onion, coarsely chopped
2 tablespoons unsalted butter
2 tablespoons red wine vinegar, divided
1 tablespoon all-purpose flour
2 tablespoons tomato paste
2 28-ounce cans whole tomatoes, preferably Muir Glen
Pinch of baking soda
1 cup water
Diamond crystal kosher salt and freshly ground black pepper, to taste
1 bay leaf
1 cup whole milk, warmed (but not boiled)
Good-tasting olive oil, to serve (optional)

In a large heavy pot, melt the butter over medium heat. When it foams, add the onion, and sauté until it softens, goes translucent, and browns a little around the edges. Add 1 tablespoon of the vinegar to deglaze the pot, scrape up the brown bits with a wooden spoon or spatula, and turn down the heat to medium-low.

Add the flour and the tomato paste, and stir to incorporate. Add the remaining tablespoon of vinegar to deglaze once again, and scrape up any flour or tomato paste that may be sticking to the pot.

Dump in the 2 cans of tomatoes and their juices and break them up a bit with a wooden spoon. (Watch out, they squirt.) Stir in the baking soda and water, season lightly with salt and pepper, add the bay leaf, partially cover, and simmer gently for about 30 minutes. Turn off the heat, remove the bay leaf, and use an immersion blender to purée the soup. (You can also carefully purée it in batches in a stand blender. As with the cream of asparagus soup on page 92, fill the blender only one-half to three-quarters of the way full with each batch. Return the puréed soup to the pot.)

Add the warmed milk very slowly, stirring constantly, just before serving. Top each bowl with a drizzle of olive oil, if you'd like, and a grind or two of black pepper.

Serves 8.

Brown Soda Bread

1¾ cups (219 grams) all-purpose flour
1¾ cups (198 grams) whole wheat flour
3 tablespoons instant oats (rolled oats chopped coarsely with a knife will also work)
1 tablespoon ground flaxseeds
2 packed tablespoons dark brown sugar
1 teaspoon baking soda
1 teaspoon fine sea salt
2 tablespoons (28 grams) cold unsalted butter, cut into ½-inch cubes, plus more for greasing the pan
2 cups buttermilk

Preheat the oven to 425 degrees and butter a 9-by-5-by-3-inch loaf pan. Combine the first seven ingredients (everything but the butter and the buttermilk) in a large bowl and blend well with a fork.

Add the butter, and rub it in with your fingertips until the mixture resembles a coarse meal. Dig a well in the center of the dry ingredients, fill with the buttermilk, and stir until the liquid is just incorporated. (Better for a bit of dry flour to remain than to overmix the dough.)

Scrape the dough into the buttered loaf pan and bake for about 35 minutes, until the crust is brown and a tester inserted into the center of the loaf comes out clean. Turn the loaf out onto a rack and cool for at least twenty minutes before slicing.

CHAPTER 31

A Funny Definition

"**W**ant to spend this summer in Berlin?" I hadn't planned on asking him just then. The thought hadn't even come to me until that moment. We were eating breakfast at our red table, the newspaper split between us. Eli looked up. Then, as casually as if I had asked him whether he'd like pizza for dinner, he said, "Sure."

A few months had gone by and I wasn't yet pregnant. I would be soon, though, I hoped. A summer in Berlin could be a last hurrah for just us two. Or maybe a first hurrah, Eli and Jess back out there, two healthy people free again to take on the world. *Hurrah!* Either way, I wanted to get out of town.

By noon we had a plan: I'd passed the German proficiency exam required by my department, but barely. If I wanted to do the comparative work I had in mind for my dissertation, I would have to improve my German. There was a summer language program in the center of Berlin. Maybe my department would pay for me to do it? It was February, which meant that summer grant applications were almost due. I completed the forms by the end of the week while Eli approached his boss about working remotely for the summer.

A few weeks later, we were set. The funding came through, permission was granted, and when we were done pinching ourselves, we started looking for a flat. It was fun, this scheming. I felt as though we were staging something not totally allowed. I couldn't wait to go.

I always remember the first picnic of the year. Probably because it feels so unlikely. All that snow and ice, months of wind-stung cheeks, pitch-black late afternoons. Then a suddenly spring day sneaks up, and there you are, with grass and a blanket and something to eat, and you slip off your jacket and you're not even cold. Like the First Day of School, First Night Sheets on laundry days, and the First Ocean Swim of the summer, First Picnic is *a thing.*

Ours was in early April that year. We'd gotten home later than expected and had to race against the sun. Eli dug the blue quilted blanket out of the bin in the hall closet. It had been his bedspread in college and for picnics ever since. I grabbed a long-sleeved shirt, and by the time we were lining up our shoes along the edge of the blanket in the park outside our apartment, it was almost a full half hour after the sun had officially set, but still another full half hour before it would be truly dark. We ate steamed artichokes, and pasta with mushrooms, lemon, and thyme. Then we stretched out on the blanket and let our conversation go where conversations go when your bellies are full and you're flat on your back outdoors, when the stars are already out but you feel like you have all night.

"People tell me I'm brave," I said. "Do you think I'm brave?"

"Do I think you're brave?" He was buying time.

"I asked you first."

"Yes," he said. "But not because you were sick. Bravery doesn't mean living through something hard."

I rolled over onto my stomach and pushed myself up on my elbows. "Say more, say better."

Eli sat up and folded himself into a cross-legged position, pulling his left heel against his body at the top of his thigh. "Bravery is when you go against the momentum of your life to do the scary thing," he began. He plucked a piece of grass and rolled it between his finger and his thumb. "So . . . okay: If a lion comes after you and backs you against a wall, and you face him, that's not brave. It's when you go after the lion yourself and stick your head into his mouth. That's brave."

"Right," I agreed. "Like, not just living through the terror, but hunting it down. It's only called bravery when you've made a choice. And that's just it. I didn't choose anything." The way I saw it, I'd just lived alongside something really bad for a while. I'd recognized that the only way out was through, and then I had waited, the way you do when you're caught in a downpour and have no choice but to get soaked until the storm clouds pass. Cowards and heroes and everyone in between would have done the same, I figured, because really, what was the alternative? I realized that I didn't know very many brave people at all, and that I wasn't nearly as brave as I wanted to be.

"You're braver than you think," Eli said.

Back inside, we opened a bottle of wine and sank into the sofa. I saw the question starting to form on Eli's lips, the same question he had been asking me for eight months now. This time, when I cut him off, he started to cry.

"You've worked so hard to get back to where you are," he said.

"You've made your body strong again. You're running. You're back in school. You are better. You are whole. But when you see that dent, you feel like you're not."

"Because I'm horrible," I said.

"Babe—"

"No, I am. If I need to fix anything, it's the thing inside of me that can't just be grateful. I know how things might have turned out. I know how they *should* have turned out. I'm supposed to be dead, Eli. *Dead.* I am lucky to have this dent."

"You have a funny definition of luck."

I bit my lip, suddenly angry. "You're wrong. Plastic surgery won't change what happened to me. It won't undo the fact that my body broke or give me back the sight in my left eye. God, what is wrong with me? Since when do I care about my looks, anyway?" I'd always been a shower-and-go person, letting my curls do whatever they pleased. At twenty-nine, a tube of lipstick was all the makeup I owned. It was the same color I'd once tried when I was sixteen from a sample tube that Amy had gotten along with a purchase. Even on my wedding day, I wore only that lipstick and a bit of eyeliner my cousin Katie brought along. I'd done my hair myself that morning, by which I mean I washed it. "It's not like I was some kind of beauty before all this," I said. "It's not like, with this dent in my head, I've lost something."

Eli closed his eyes. "It hurts me to hear you talk about yourself this way."

"I'm sorry. I'm so sorry, love. You didn't sign up for this." Now I was crying, too.

"*You* didn't sign up for this. And you can't move past it if every time you look in the mirror, you're reminded of it. You shouldn't have to remember it all the time."

"You don't solve problems with plastic surgery," I insisted.

Eli gathered my feet onto his lap. "It's not that kind of plastic surgery." His tone had changed. He was no longer pleading. "All you want is to look the way you did. To recognize yourself in the mirror again."

I felt tired. I didn't know what to say. I crawled over to his side of the sofa and laid my head on his chest, dent side down. He swept his hand across my back.

"I'm going to make an appointment with the surgeon," he said. "If you want to, you can cancel it."

I didn't cancel it. The doctor walked into the examining room and around to the dented side of my head.

"I can fix that," he said. Just like that. Like a mechanic looking at a bent fender. He would go in along the old incision line, peel my forehead back down, and fill my remaining hole with something called methyl methacrylate, a hot putty that hardens as it cools. I asked if the reconstruction would take care of the remaining tenderness and discomfort, but he couldn't say. I hesitated.

"I need more time," I told Eli, and I could have it. The OR was booked for months. We were leaving soon to spend Memorial Day weekend with my family in Ohio. Maybe they could help me figure this out. I could think about it while we were away in Berlin, and by the end of the summer, maybe, *maybe* I could be ready.

I was in the kitchen at my dad and Amy's house when the phone call came in: There was an unexpected opening in the doctor's schedule on June 9. If I wanted the surgery, I could have that slot.

"You mean, twelve days from now?" I asked the secretary.

"Yes."

The doctor knew about our planned trip to Berlin, that we were leaving at the end of the month. I'd have three weeks between the surgery and our departure, and he said I'd be recovered enough to make the trip.

My brain switched into solve-it mode.

"Okay," I said, getting my bearings. "Thank you. I'll need to speak with my husband, call the insurance company . . ."

"Oh, they'll cover it," she said. "If they cover reconstructive surgery, which I bet they do."

I paused. "This is reconstructive surgery?" I hadn't thought of it that way.

"Certainly. You know, like breast reconstruction after mastectomy. It's like that. To make you look like you did before you got sick."

Eli had said essentially the same thing, but those words, "reconstructive surgery" changed something for me. If a woman who'd survived cancer wanted her body to look as it once had, I'd think it was only natural. I remembered a conversation I'd had with Rebecca, who, years after predicting the union of Eli and Jess, had continued to be smart about everything. She was someone I called when I needed a gut check, a little help knowing what I likely already knew. I was sure she'd be with me in the no-more-surgery camp. She wasn't. "It's your fucking face, Jessica," she'd said.

My family felt the same. They were so careful, so sensitive about respecting whatever I chose that they hesitated to offer any advice. I had to ask a bunch of times. Finally, around the table in the yard, after a dinner of grilled burgers, pickles, and extra mustard for me, Amy said, "I'd do it, if it were my face. Absolutely." I looked at my dad.

"Absolutely," he repeated.

The next night, our friends Janet and Fred came over for dinner. I'd turned thirty that week, and Janet brought cake. It was white through and through, made with coconut milk and swathed in cream cheese frosting. Someone lit the candles and put the cake down on the table in front of me, and my father took a photo with an old Polaroid camera. It's a black-and-white photo on the kind of film that you have to peel apart to get to the developed image. The room was dark, so the photo is mostly black, but the glow of the cake is bright and lights up my hands and a part of my face—the intact part. The dent in my head is in a shadow, and you can't see it at all.

The nurse in the recovery room handed me a mirror. I remember pausing to shove any expectation down to the bottom of me. Then I lifted the mirror and looked. What I saw there, I can hardly tell you. I was completely unprepared. I had asked for the mirror so that I could look at "it." At the dent, or the former site of the dent, or whatever it would be. But when I peered into the glass, I saw something else instead: my face. I saw *me*. A me I hadn't seen since early on the morning of August 19, 2008, when I had pulled my hair back into a ponytail and laced up my running shoes in front of the mirror in my hotel room. "Hey!" I wanted to shout. "I know you! I've been trying to get ahold of you for ages! Where on earth have you been?!"

I had completely underestimated the power of that dent in my head. For almost two years, I had done whatever I could to force my eye away from the broken parts. When I would look in the mirror, I would search my cheeks, my jawline, my lips, for signs of the face I had known. Sometimes, for a split second, I would find it, but then that dent would pull my eye right back. It might as well have been a giant blanket cloaking my entire face. That's when I got it: It wasn't seeing the defect, but *not* seeing *me* that had torn me apart all those months. In that recovery room, even with the swelling beginning to creep in, there was nothing to distract me from the person staring back at me. It was so good to see her. I was grateful to have found her. I didn't want to look away.

Janet's Coconut Cake

The cake that I know as Janet's is actually an Ina Garten recipe to which Janet made one small, brilliant change. Instead of whole milk, Janet uses coconut milk in the batter. Thanks to the added fat, you end up with an especially rich and tender crumb. Be careful at the store not to pick up "coconut milk beverage" or "coconut milk drink," which are thin and watery. You're looking for pure coconut milk in a can. You don't have to be a die-hard coconut lover to enjoy this cake, by the way. The coconut flavor is nice and gentle.

Janet adapted this recipe from Ina Garten's *Barefoot Contessa at Home*.

For the cake:

  1½ cups (3 sticks; 340 grams) unsalted butter, at cool room temperature, plus more for greasing the pans
  2 cups (400 grams) granulated sugar
  6 large eggs, at room temperature
  1½ teaspoons pure vanilla extract
  1½ teaspoons pure almond extract
  3 cups (375 grams) all-purpose flour, plus more for dusting the pans
  1 teaspoon baking powder
  ½ teaspoon baking soda
  ½ teaspoon fine sea salt
  1 cup well-shaken coconut milk
  1¼ cup (113 grams) shredded unsweetened coconut

For the frosting:

> 1 pound (454 grams) cream cheese, at room temperature
>
> 1 cup (2 sticks; 226 grams) unsalted butter, at room temperature
>
> 1 teaspoon pure vanilla extract
>
> ¼ teaspoon pure almond extract
>
> 3½ cups (454 grams) confectioners' sugar, sifted
>
> 1¾ cup (165 grams) shredded unsweetened coconut, for finishing

Bake the cakes:

Preheat the oven to 350 degrees. Butter two round 9-inch cake pans, then line the bottoms with cut-out circles of parchment paper. Butter the paper, and lightly dust with flour.

In the bowl of a stand mixer fitted with the paddle attachment, cream the 1½ cups butter and the granulated sugar on medium speed for 3 to 5 minutes, until fluffy. Crack the eggs into a glass. With the mixer on medium speed, add the eggs one at a time, waiting for each egg to be fully incorporated before slipping the next one in. Pause to scrape down the bowl after mixing in the third egg, then again once all of the eggs have been incorporated. Add the 1½ teaspoons each of vanilla and almond extract, and mix well. It's okay if the mixture looks curdled.

In a separate bowl, sift together the flour, baking powder, baking soda, and salt. With the mixer on low speed, add half of the dry ingredients, then all of the coconut milk, then the rest of the dry ingredients. Mix until just combined. Fold in the 4 ounces coconut with a rubber spatula.

Pour the batter into the prepared pans and spread evenly. Bake for 40 to 50 minutes, until the tops are brown and a toothpick inserted into the centers comes out clean. Cool in their pans on a rack for 30 minutes, then turn the cakes out onto the rack and cool completely.

Make the frosting:

Put the cream cheese, the 1 cup butter, the 1 teaspoon vanilla, and the ¼ teaspoon almond extract in the bowl of a stand mixer fitted with the paddle attachment. Add the confectioners' sugar and continue mixing on low speed, just until smooth. Do not whip.

Assemble the cake:

Tear four 2- to 3-inch strips of wax paper and arrange them in a square on your cake stand or serving plate. Place one cake layer, top side down, in the center of the square, with the four strips of wax paper partially sticking out on all sides. (The strips are to keep the plate clean from frosting. You'll remove them before serving, taking any smears with you.)

Spread the top of the cake layer with frosting. Place the second layer on top, top side up, and frost the entire cake. Sprinkle with coconut and lightly press some onto the sides, then remove the wax paper. Serve at room temperature.

Serves 12.

CHAPTER 32

Move Along Now

Our Berlin flat on Prenzlauer Allee was in a building painted marigold yellow. Bright pennant flag bunting ran across the sidewalk between a lamppost and the awning of the shop downstairs. The neighborhood, Prenzlauer Berg, once part of East Berlin, was a mix of small businesses and residences, with a tramline running through it down our street. At the stop across from our building, you could board the M2 and be in the center of town in eight minutes. My German classes were there, at the Goethe-Institut on Neue Schönhauser Strasse. I would often walk home. When I'd spot the flags flapping in the breeze, I'd know I was almost there.

I had found our flat on craigslist—rather the flat had found us, when a woman named Olivia responded to our listing. Olivia would be traveling all summer with her boyfriend, Fabian, and they were looking for subletters, and would their flat perhaps meet our needs? "Greetings," she signed off at the end of her e-mail.

It was a modest flat comprising a small bedroom and a larger space divided into a living room and an eat-in kitchen. All the windows stretched from floor to ceiling and swung open to shallow Juliet balconies, except for in the living room, where they opened onto an actual balcony on the back of the building. There was a little table out there, two chairs, and a few potted plants that I'd do my best not to kill. Below was a brick and cement patio, and just beyond it, a yard of tall grass, trees, wildflowers, and vines. In the mornings, light filtered through the foliage and cast leafy shadows on the hardwood floors.

On the other side of the apartment, the bedroom looked out over the square courtyard and entryway. We slept with the window open and awoke to the early morning sounds of our neighbors: a man singing, a child's voice, someone's daily coughing fit. Two stories up, a disembodied mannequin leg stuck straight out into the courtyard between the balcony bars. I knew it wasn't real, but I always looked twice.

We had landed in Berlin three weeks postsurgery. I was at that curious stage of recovery that feels less like fading illness and more like persistent, low-grade disorientation, when you neither trust in the absolute health of your own body nor completely dismiss it. It is not unlike the disorientation one feels when living in a new city, speaking a new language, finding one's footing in a new routine, swinging wildly between the certainty that you are doing fine and the certainty that you are not. My first few weeks in Berlin, I wasn't always sure if it was the new head on my shoulders or the new ground beneath my feet that had me feeling at once tilted and tired, giddy and at times quite faint. It was probably a little of both. I chose to think of it as the latter.

Berlin is beautiful in a rough-around-the-edges kind of way. You can see the seams between the old and the new, between the new and the newer, and I like that. Eli and I had been in Berlin together once before in college, when our choir went on a spring break tour through Germany. We spent only a couple of days in Berlin, but it made an impression. This was over a year before we started dating, yet I remember both of us saying that we wanted to spend some more time there.

Now we had a whole summer to get to know the city. We could do all the tourist stuff and still have plenty of time for very important things like finding a favorite breakfast spot, learning never to stand in the bicycle lane while waiting for the light to change, and cultivating opinions about the best yogurts and breads to be had; time for walking directly from the tram station to the supermarket after spotting a chocolate-dipped rice cake, something called a *Schoko Reiswaffel*, in the hands of a little boy on the M2. It was fun to dig in and really live there, to buy sunflower seed bread, *Sonnen-blumenkernbrot*, by the loaf, slice and toast it in our own kitchen in our own toaster, and slather it with plum butter or quark; to sit on the balcony with a bowlful of fresh red currants, pluck them from their stems or pop them off with our teeth, and feel them burst on our tongues, like sweet-and-sour caviar.

We visited the Pergamon, the Hamburger Bahnhof, and what's left of the wall at Mauerpark, but we also hosted new friends for dinner, washed piles of dishes, and negotiated the return of an Internet router in a language that's not our own. We walked miles. Sometimes with soft, warm pretzels in hand, sometimes clutching tiny cups of hazelnut gelato and even tinier spoons.

My classes were in the afternoons, so mornings were mine. I'd carry my German workbook down the street to Café Anna Blume, order a black tea with milk and a croissant with apricot-sage jam, and do my homework. On the weekends, Eli would join me. We'd order a multitiered platter of fruit, cheese, sugared crepes, fresh rolls, and smoked fish, and settle in for two hours.

A few blocks from our flat, past the stationery shop with the pretty paper notebooks, the dusty paper lanterns that hung in a storefront window, the baby boutique with the Marimekko bibs, and the bakery with the disappointing pastries, a farmers' market set up twice a week. We had arrived in Berlin in the middle of a heat wave that kept us from cooking much at first. We stuck with mostly stovetop and cutting board meals: eggs and rice, sautéed zucchini with plum sauce, heaps of strawberries for dessert. But the surest way to make a home feel like home is to turn on the oven, so when the heat finally broke, I squeezed through the market crowd, picked up a basket of apricots, and plotted my first bake.

I worked without a recipe, rubbing a block of butter into flour, sugar, and oats until I'd formed a topping that was more dough than crumble. The consistency was wetter and heavier than my usual mixture, but instead of adding more flour or oats, I decided to leave it alone. I halved the apricots and arranged them in a baking dish, then buried them under the topping. It was so thick that I had to spread it with a spoon and sort of pat it into place. Just out of the oven I could see it was something special. The apricots had brightened in color and flavor and melted into rich, almost spreadable versions of themselves. The top was like a sprawling oatmeal cookie.

I made it again for dinner guests a few days later, which left me with three apricots, too few for a crumble or a pie. So I halved them, removed the pits, dredged them in sugar, and set them in a baking dish. There was an open bottle of white wine on the counter that I emptied into the dish to form a shallow pool around the apricots, just enough to cover their bottoms, and cooked them in a hot oven. A half hour later, the wine was now a syrup. The apricots had gone all bold and buttery as apricots do. They looked heavy, full, crinkled around the edges, as though waking up from a deep sleep.

I took out two cereal bowls and spooned an apricot and a half and some of the winey syrup into each one while Eli grabbed the vanilla ice cream for on top. We went out to the balcony, to the little table and chairs, and I sat down, drew my knees up to my chin, and took a bite.

Where I sat on that balcony in Berlin with a bowl of baked apricots resting on my knees was where I might have sat had I never been sick at all. It felt that way sometimes, as though the aneurysm had never happened, as though by living through it to the other side, I'd arrived somewhere that felt conspicuously, gloriously, like where and who I'd once been. At the same time, not at all.

I had tried to resist the idea of a before and an after. I was adamant that in all those long months of illness and recovery, nothing had changed, least of all me. To admit change was to admit defeat, I thought, to concede that I had allowed myself to be carried off by the current of this terrible thing.

But we are always swept this way and that. We create the life we want to live, yes. Then, in return, that life creates us. We follow the tides; we have no choice. We splash about beneath the brightest of moons, then the darkest of skies, tug hard from the surface on anchors that refuse to budge, and then, if we are very brave, dive deep. There in Berlin, I felt it: Things *were* different. *I* was different. And what's more, I didn't want to go back to the way things were before.

* * *

The plastic surgeon had said there was no reason to wait, so we didn't, and three weeks into our Berlin stay I realized I was late. I stood alone in the bathroom for a minute disbelieving, staring at the dark blue lines, then ran into the bedroom and tackled Eli at his desk.

It occurred to me that night as I was falling asleep that I must have believed on some level that I could have only one or the other, a fixed head or a child. Because all I could think of now was, *I get to have both.* The timing felt perfect and a bit like magic. A successful surgery, then right away, this?

I didn't want my pregnancy to feel like any kind of redemption—that was way too heavy a burden for a child to bear. But I couldn't help but imagine sometimes that conception was a peace offering from my body to me, as though we were separate, or had been, and were calling a truce. *My body is doing this!* I'd think. *Not so broken after all!* I rushed to claim my physical self in a way I never had before. I didn't marvel at the miracle of pregnancy as much as I reveled in its normalcy. *Nothing to see here, folks, move along now. Just MAKING A BABY UNDER MY SHIRT.*

It was all wonderfully elastic, the way Eli and I hadn't wanted children and then we did, the way I'd been healthy, then sick, and now healthy again. That after all that had happened, my life could snap back into shape, just a bit stretched out here and there—it felt impossible, and also only natural. Sometime in March, a new human would be here.

Megan was scheduled to arrive during my last week of classes. The three of us would be off to Prague for the weekend, after which Eli and I would travel on to St. Petersburg and Amsterdam before a final few days in Berlin. We hadn't told anyone about the pregnancy except for my mom, but we were planning on sharing the news with Megan. With nausea beginning to set in and so much time together coming up, we didn't see any way around it, and in any case, we were excited to get to say it out loud to our best friend.

We'd been tracking Megan's flight and knew she had landed. She'd be at our place any minute. "Do you want to say it, or should I?" I asked Eli as I ran to the bathroom. I couldn't wait to see my friend.

Something red. I saw it before I saw it. My brain needed a sec to catch up.

"No," I said out loud to no one.

Eli looked up an obstetrician and I got on the phone with a receptionist who spoke no English. I didn't have the words I needed in German, so I did my best and hoped to be understood:

"Ich habe keine Kinder, aber ich werde vielleicht im März ein Kind haben, und ich habe jetzt viel Blut gesehen." I don't have any children, but maybe in March I will, and I have just seen a lot of blood. The doctor saw me right away, and by the following week, it was done. Meanwhile, Megan left for Prague without us.

The doctor had been gentle and kind. There was some comic relief thanks to our language issues. "Hmm . . . you know . . . Michael Jackson, mm-hm? Bye-bye, Michael Jackson?" he said when trying to communicate what they would use to anesthetize me during the procedure. "Ven you have hemorrhage . . . hm . . . lots of Blut, mm-hm? You vill go in hospital." It took me a beat to realize that by "ven" he meant not the English word "when," but the German *wenn,* "if." (I watched the color return to Eli's face as I explained as much.)

We went in for a follow-up appointment right before we flew home. The doctor sat us down at his desk, pushed his patient notebook over to me, and thumbed through it quickly, like a flipbook.

There were colored dots by many of the names. A blue dot meant one miscarriage, a yellow dot meant two, a red dot meant three or more, he explained. Almost every one of these women, he said, is now a mother.

I nodded, numbly. He told me that as many as one in four pregnancies ends in miscarriage, that having a miscarriage didn't mean I was at any greater risk for another. He urged me to see this as a good thing. Sperm was meeting egg. This was excellent news. It was only a matter of time.

I wanted to find comfort in what he was saying, but all I could think was that this was proof. My body *was* broken. It was. I'd been foolish to think otherwise. *Of course I'm not supposed to reproduce. I'm not supposed to be here at all.*

I spoke with my gynecologist at home. "I know things are hard now," she said, "but soon, they will be perfect."

Baked Apricots with Cardamom Pistachios

You'll end up with more vanilla sugar than you need for this recipe. Save what's left in a lidded jar for sprinkling on cinnamon toast, whipping into cream, or stirring into anything that might benefit from a hint of vanilla flavor. If you'd rather not splurge on the vanilla bean, ½ teaspoon of vanilla extract will do. As for the white wine, use whatever you have on hand. I've tried everything from Moscato d'Asti to sauvignon blanc with splendid results. I don't think you can go wrong.

Serve these warm, with a pour of cold sweet cream or a scoop of vanilla ice cream if you'd like, though they don't need it. I store the leftovers in a jar in the fridge and eat them chilled over yogurt or oatmeal. My friend Carrie puts them on a sandwich with melted cheese. That sounds like a plan to me.

½ cup white wine
1 cup (200 grams) granulated sugar
1 vanilla bean
8 apricots, halved and pitted
⅓ cup (45 grams) shelled, roasted, and salted pistachios
1–2 pinches ground cardamom

Heat the oven to 425 degrees.

Pour the wine into a 2½-quart baking dish. (Swirl in the vanilla extract, if using.) Put the sugar into a bowl, split the vanilla bean with a sharp knife, scrape out the seeds, and rub them into the sugar with your fingertips. Measure 3 to 4 tablespoons of the sugar into a shallow bowl or pie plate. Transfer the remaining sugar to an airtight jar, bury the scraped-out vanilla pod inside, and reserve for another time.

Press the apricot halves into the sugar to coat them on both sides, then place them, skin side down, in the wine bath. Bake for 35 to 40 minutes, until the apricots have deepened in color, puckered around the edges, and barely resist when you poke them with a fork. Meanwhile, coarsely chop the pistachios and toss them with the cardamom.

To serve, spoon a few warm apricots and a bit of the winey syrup into each bowl, and scatter with a spoonful of nuts.

Serves 4.

CHAPTER 33

Any Day

Prune plums were back in the market. September is their time. I spotted them in the far bin and stepped carefully through the crowd. We'd been home from Berlin for a year. That spring, we'd moved from our one-bedroom apartment into the larger unit next door. We had a proper dining room now, with space for a proper table. Our small red one was now my writing desk. From our living room and bedroom windows, I could see the park. There was our picnic spot, the playground, the field.

I picked up a plum and ran my thumb across its cloudy purple skin. Prune plums are more oval than round, egglike, only smaller. When you hold one in the palm of your hand and close your fingers around it, it all but disappears.

"Taste one," the farmer said. "I'd say taste two, but I assume you guys can share." He winked, gesturing at my belly. I smiled and bit into the fruit's flesh, sweet-tart and firm. "When are you due?" he asked.

"Any day," I said and felt a ripple beneath my ribs, as though on cue. The sugar from the plum had reached her fast. I walked home, my tote bulging with plums, bumping gently against my hip.

Prune plums are nice enough straight from the tree, but really, they're for cooking. Heat emboldens them. They hold their form beautifully in the oven and emerge plump with juices, deep purple and sweet. I'd never thought of plum as a flavor, distinct and retrievable from my memory like green apple, banana, or peach. Then I tasted a prune plum, cooked—baked, actually, into a buttery cake— and thought, *I know what a plum tastes like now.*

I put a cut-up stick of butter into a pot and swirled it over a low flame. Then in went the sugar, the vanilla and almond extracts, the flour, and the salt. I popped one hip, steering my belly to the side so that I could move in closer, stirred the mixture into a soft dough, and pressed it into a fluted pan.

As the crust baked, I tipped the plums onto the counter, washed and dried them, cut them lengthwise down their center seams, and pulled them apart. I had a plum half in one hand, the pit I'd just pried loose in the other, when I felt a now-familiar ache in my back, an insistent tightening around my middle. Still holding the fruit, I leaned over the counter on folded arms and breathed deeply until the tension released. These contractions were just practice. I'd been feeling them for weeks.

The crust in the oven darkened a shade. The scent of almond and butter hit. Of cakes, of cookies, of macaroons, of gratitude for where I'd been and where I was going. I felt the desire to nourish and be nourished, to make something, to *be* something. The desire to begin.

On September 9, 2011, our daughter came screaming out into the world. Nine days later, in a living room full of our family and closest friends, we named her: Mia Louise, after my grandmothers. Julia and Eitan brought cupcakes; my sister Kasey brought bagels. There was lox and champagne and fruit. I didn't cook a thing.

Megan had flown in from Los Angeles for the gathering and after everyone had left she pulled out a gift.

"For Mia," she said. "I hope you like it."

I unwound the tissue paper from around something hard, narrow, and flat, about the length of a shoe box: a wooden ramp. And an elephant, painted blue, that rocked its way down, *ke-donk, ke-donk, ke-donk*. We stood there watching it go, Megan, Eli, and I, with a snoozing Mia in my arms.

"Megan!" I was delighted. "Where did you find this?"

"Prague," she said.

It took me a second to understand what she was saying, for the trip she had made without us to come to mind.

"That was more than a year ago."

"Yeah," Megan said. "I've been holding on to it for her."

"But . . . How . . . ?" I didn't know what to say.

Megan smiled. "I knew she'd come."

Once-upon-a-times have a way of sneaking up on you. Stories never begin where they begin. Mia was stirring. With her eyes still closed she moved her head side to side, nuzzling into my chest. "Hi, sweetheart," I whispered into her ear. I sat down on the sofa, laid her on my lap with her head up by my knees, and stroked her tiny fists. She smacked her lips and poked her tongue out, searching, hungry. I drew her to my breast, and she ate.

Italian Prune Plum Tart

Italian prune plums arrive in the final weeks of summer and don't stick around for long, so when you see them, grab them and make this tart. The press-in crust keeps things simple and bakes up beautifully into a sweet and salty shortbread-like shell. Then all that's left to do is fill it with fruit, whisk together a custard, pour it over top, and bake. While I'm waiting for prune plums to come around, I make this with apricots, instead. Delicious.

For the pastry:

1¼ cups plus 1 tablespoon (180 grams) all-purpose flour

½ teaspoon sea salt flakes, like Maldon

½ cup (1 stick; 113 grams) unsalted butter, melted and cooled

½ cup (100 grams) granulated sugar

¼ teaspoon pure almond extract

¼ teaspoon pure vanilla extract

For the filling:

½ cup heavy whipping cream

1 large egg, lightly beaten

½ teaspoon pure vanilla extract

3 tablespoons granulated sugar

1 tablespoon flour

10–13 Italian prune plums, pitted and halved

Heat the oven to 350 degrees and generously butter the bottom and sides of a 9-inch fluted tart pan with a removable bottom.

Make the pastry:

Whisk together the flour and salt in a medium bowl, and set aside. Put the sugar and melted butter into a large bowl and mix well with a spoon. Add the extracts, flour, and salt to the sugar and butter mixture, and stir to form a soft dough. Transfer the dough to the center of the buttered pan and press it evenly into the bottom and sides of the pan. Bake for 13 to 15 minutes, until the dough puffs slightly and takes on a bit of color. Set aside to cool. (It doesn't need to cool all the way to room temperature, just enough so that you won't cook the egg in the custard on contact.)

While the pastry is baking, make the custard:

Whisk together the flour and sugar in a small bowl. Combine the heavy cream, egg, and vanilla in a medium bowl, and whisk well. Add the flour and sugar, and whisk again until smooth.

Place the prune plums cut-side down into the cooled pastry in two concentric circles, with one in the center. Pour the custard into the tart around the fruit. Bake for 40 to 45 minutes, until the custard is just set and the top blushes with spots of golden brown. Cool before serving.

Serves 8 to 10.

Acknowledgments

This book would not exist had I not been around to write it. To all of my doctors in Burlington and Boston who diagnosed me, took me apart, fixed what was broken, and put me back together again: Thank you for saving my life.

I am especially grateful to Dr. Bruce Tranmer for his intelligence and warmth, for never losing sight of the person in the patient, and for assembling and mentoring a team of brilliant residents who practice medicine with great courage, compassion, and humility.

At Fletcher Allen, I was fortunate to be in the hands of extraordinary nurses and aides, generous, unflinching souls who kept me feeling human in my darkest hours. They were my world. In flipping through an old notebook from my hospital stay, I found a list in my father's handwriting with the heading "Nurses We Love." Susan Amidon, Carolina Baldwin, Greg Brooks, Erin Charles, Peter Clark, Patty Crease, Amela Dulma, Aimee Eaton, Darlene Fraize, Mike Higgins, Pete Kassel, M. J. McMahon, and Michelle Norse: Thank you for your care.

One terrifying night in the emergency department back in Boston, I met a young doctor named Kristopher Kahle. He acted as my advocate and ally, above the call of duty. Thank you, Dr. Kahle, for making me feel less alone, and for helping a girl get some Tylenol.

I am grateful to all who helped me settle back into my body once the gravest danger had passed. Jeffrey Fergerson got me moving again in the earliest days of my recovery and let me talk his ear off about food on our many laps around the rehab center. Aimee Klein picked up where Jeff left off, pushing me with humor and resolve to trust in my own strength. And where would I be without Holly Herman? Holly is a force who practices physical therapy with the utmost generosity and skill. She told me that pain is temporary—and proved it.

To all my dear friends mentioned in this book, and the many who are not: Thank you for your every kindness, for guiding me through, and keeping me sane. You made me whole again.

If the food in this book is delicious, it's because I had help from some first-rate bakers and cooks. Alana Chernila let me pick her brain about recipe writing (among many other things). Ashley Rodriguez helped me get my plum tart just right. René Becker entrusted me with his almond macaroon recipe and helped me adapt it for the home kitchen. Andrew Janjigian was endlessly generous with his knowledge of all things flour, yeast, and beyond. Molly Birnbaum edited my recipes with care and, together with Andrew, spent a dizzying amount of time discussing measurements, leaveners, pie crusts—anything and everything that kept me up at night about telling people what to do in their kitchens.

My neighbors Cansu Canca, Holger Spamann, April Paffrath, Matthew Krom, Esmé Krom, Sam and Elisha Gechter, Lisa Ceglia, Andrew Blom, and Cecilia Blom came through with spare eggs, sticks of butter, cups of milk, and more during recipe testing when my own kitchen came up short. Sam and Elisha let me stuff them silly with many rounds of cookies, cakes, breads, and pies. They gave me their honest reviews so that I could do better.

To my recipe testers, Marco Ajello, Katie Baxter, Talya Benoff, Molly Birnbaum, Andrew Blom, Carrie Bornstein, Alana Chernila, Stephanie Cornell, Amy Fechtor, Anna Fechtor, Kasey Fechtor, Rivka Friedman, Lynn Glickman, Sarit Kattan Gribetz, Janet Helgeson, Hannah Heller, Eitan Hersh, Julia Hoffman, Esmé Krom, Isabelle Levy, Becky Lurie, Laurie Mazur, Lisa Moussalli, Sandra Naddaff, April Paffrath, Adena Silberstein, Amy Thompson, Lukas Volger, and Kit Wannen: a from-the-rooftops thank-you for your many hours in the kitchen, your attention to detail, your very fine taste, your thoughtful, thorough feedback, and your enthusiasm for this project.

One million thanks and at least as many cookies are due to the people in my life who have helped me to write:

To the readers of Sweet Amandine, for your kindness and companionship, for believing in what the kitchen has to tell us, and in me. When I got stuck along the way, I'd think of all of you, remember for whom I was writing, and carry on.

To my sixth grade teacher Deb Delisle, who made a special place for me beneath the spider plant to sit and write.

To my high school English teachers Nancy Brunswick, Bob Hastings, and Jan Morgan, for teaching me how to think about words on a page. Of the many competing voices in my head when I write, yours are ones I listen to.

To Savine Weizman, for long talks on Saturday afternoons, for introducing me to Rilke, for your profound understanding of what it means to strive in writing and in life, and for broccoli with mayonnaise.

To my fellow students in Darcy Frey's creative nonfiction seminar, for helping me see that there was a story here, and encouraging me to tell it.

To the faculty, staff, and alumni of the Wexner Graduate Fellowship for standing by me, for caring about this project, and supporting me in every way.

To my new friends and colleagues at the Makeshift Society, and to Shannon Lehman, for softening the landing when I moved with my family to San Francisco in the final weeks of this project, and seeing me through to the finish.

To Professor Ruth Wisse, for your wise counsel over the years, for cheering me on at every turn, for reminding me that while life is short, it is also long, and for encouraging me to write.

To Eitan Kensky, a brilliant writer and friend, for your support and confidence in me.

To Steve Jacobson, for seeing me so clearly and believing in me.

To Mary Medlin, for caring about stories and how they're told, for your faith in me, and for your friendship.

To Molly Wizenberg and Luisa Weiss, for paving the way, for boosting me up, and for so much inspiration—plus plenty of nuts-and-bolts advice and even some saving the day.

To Eitan Hersh, Julia Hoffman, Sarit Kattan Gribetz, and Jonathan Gribetz, for your enduring friendship, for knowing me well and loving me anyway, for being so damn smart, and for your clear-eyed feedback on my proposal and manuscript.

To Molly Birnbaum, whom I've already mentioned twice, but it isn't enough: for your hands-on help with every single stage of this project, for your wisdom and your cheers, and what feels like a lifetime of friendship over the past five years.

I am fortunate to have landed at Penguin with this book-to-be three years ago. Caroline Sutton saw in this project everything I hoped it would be and granted me the time and space to get the job done. Lavina Lee patiently awaited the final manuscript and worked her magic to get everything just right. Thanks to Sheila Moody for her smart and thorough copyediting, to Liz Byer for her meticulous proofreading, and to Matthew Daddona for helping to shepherd this first-time author through the sometimes confusing publishing process.

To Lindsay Gordon, Casey Maloney, and Farin Schlussel, thank you for getting behind this book so fully, and for calming my nerves as we released it into the world. I also benefited greatly from the insights of Hillary Tisman and Nach Waxman on what happens to a book once the writing is done. Thanks to you both for sharing your considerable wisdom.

I was still several thousand words and many pages of revisions from the finish line when I first saw the cover design for this book. My energy was flagging, but Alison Forner's beautiful work inspired me to finish strong and create a final product that would deliver what her cover promises. I am also grateful to Eve Kirch for an interior design that reflects the spirit and tone of this book.

My editor, Becky Cole, can hold an entire book in her head at once and flip through it as though the pages were right in front of her. For editing so smart it felt like cheating, for dazzling me with her flare for structure and form, for her patience, her humor, and for taking such good care of me and this book, I am unspeakably grateful.

My agent, Rebecca Friedman, always knows just what to do. Thank you, friend, for being right about everything, for having my back, for your intelligence and intuition about what makes a story sing, for getting this book into Becky's hands, right where it belonged, and for not marrying Eli.

To my writing partner Katrina Goldsaito, who dove deep into

the mud with me and stayed until every word was in place: What can I say? Without you, this book would not be this book. For your x-ray vision, for keeping me true, for the courage to find my voice and use it, for inspiring me with your own brilliant, sparkling prose, for our weekly meetings and countless e-mails, phone calls, and texts that kept me afloat, thank you. I can't wait for more.

To Megan Metcalf, for that luminous mind of yours and oversized heart, for seeing me, for lifting me up, for letting us claim you as family, for suggesting I start Sweet Amandine, and introducing me to Katrina; for the wooden bird from Prague you saved in secret for years because you had a feeling there would be two, and for presenting it to our Freddie when she came along. I'm so grateful for you, friend.

My cousin Katie Wannen knows what's what. She enriched this story with her insights on illness and recovery, and my life with her intelligence and grace. Thank you to my great-aunt Eileen Farkas, my grandfather Robert Fechtor, and Jill Brock for always asking about my writing, for being so smart and so good, and for their faith in me. I wrote many of these pages with my grandmother Louise Fechtor, of blessed memory, in mind. I hope she shines in them.

Yeseny Alvarez isn't family, but she might as well be. For your energy and smarts, for delighting my daughters, for loving them as if they were your own, and playing no small role making them the wonderful creatures they are; for teaching me by example how to be the parent I want to be, thank you. I would still be on chapter one, Yeseny, if it weren't for you.

Thank you to my sisters- and brothers-in-law, Jonathan Schleifer, Katie Connolly, Yitzchak Schleifer, Talya Benoff, and Atara Schleifer for their support and love throughout my recovery and the writing of this book. Special thanks to Katie for her insight and encouragement at the earliest stages of this project. And to Leslie Rosenberg, for being a kindred spirit.

To Sarah and Steve Schleifer, thank you for Eli, and for you, for welcoming me into your family from day one and showing me the kind of love parents usually reserve for their own flesh and blood. Thank you, Sarah, for teaching me more than you know about family and love. Thank you, Steve, for taking an interest in my work, and for our many important conversations throughout the creation of this book. I love the way you think.

I am grateful to my brother and sisters, Caleb Fechtor, Kasey Fechtor, and Anna Fechtor, for their discerning eyes, their excellent taste, and for inspiring me with their own writing, baking, and art. Your support means the world to me. Thank you, Caleb, for your patience with me when this book and new motherhood kept me from making it across the river as often as I would have liked; to Kasey, for hours upon hours of hanging out with your nieces so that I could sit and write; and to Anna, for three weeks of tremendous help with the girls as I found my way back to this project after Freddie was born.

My parents taught me that I could be anything, which was convenient when, at age thirty-one, I decided to try to write a book.

To my mother, Laurie Mazur: Thank you for understanding me completely, for your careful eye and intelligent notes that helped me tame and tighten this narrative, and for dropping everything time and again to fly in and save the day.

Thank you to my father, Stephen Fechtor, for knowing exactly how to be and what to say, and to my stepmother, Amy Thompson, for showing me how it's done.

To my daughters, Mia and Freddie: Thank you for being you.

And to Eli: Thank you for your love. We're just getting started.

About the Author

Jessica Fechtor writes the popular food blog Sweet Amandine. She is a PhD candidate in Jewish literature at Harvard University and lives with her husband and daughters in San Francisco.